AF901532

Pet Owner Educational Atlas

Cats

edra

Copyright © 2021 Grupo Asís Biomedia, SL
Plaza Antonio Beltrán Martínez n.° 1, planta 8 - letra I
(Centro empresarial El Trovador)
50002 Zaragoza - Spain

First printing: September 2021

This book was originally published in Spanish under the title:
Atlas de Información al Propietario: especie felina 2.ª ed.
© 2021 Grupo Asís Biomedia, SL
ISBN Spanish edition: 978-84-18339-51-6

Translation:
Owen Howard

Illustrators:
Jacob Gragera Artal
Paula Marco Peinado

ISBN: 978-84-18498-26-8
DL: Z 1364-2021

Design, layout and printing:
Grupo Asís Biomedia, SL
www.grupoasis.com
info@grupoasis.com

GRUPO asis

edra is an imprint of Grupo Asís

All rights reserved.

Any form of reproduction, distribution, publication or transformation of this book is only permitted with the authorisation of its copyright holders, apart from the exceptions allowed by law. Contact CEDRO (Spanish Centre of Reproduction Rights, www.cedro.org) if you need to photocopy or scan any part of this book (www.conlicencia.com; 0034 91 702 19 70/0034 93 272 04 47).

Warning:

Veterinary science is constantly evolving, as are pharmacology and the other sciences. Inevitably, it is therefore the responsibility of the veterinary surgeon to determine and verify the dosage, the method of administration, the duration of treatment and any possible contraindications to the treatments given to each individual patient, based on his or her professional experience. Neither the publisher nor the author can be held liable for any damage or harm caused to people, animals or properties resulting from the correct or incorrect application of the information contained in this book.

PROLOGUE

Since it was published, the first edition of this Atlas has been something I use daily in my practice. Allowing the owners could see, and above all understand, the disease affecting their cat proven essential in providing clients with explanations on everything from new diagnostic procedures to the treatments prescribed to their pet.

Why a new edition? Feline medicine is constantly changing. For this reason it was important to update this atlas accordingly. This second edition includes new guides for the assessment of acute and chronic pain, which are essential to monitor the patient in the consultation or when hospitalised, and to teach the owner to recognise pain at home. Urology is a particularly important field in feline medicine, and we have added new material to explain the treatment of ureteral obstructions using new procedures such as SUB (subcutaneous ureteral bypass). The chapters on dentistry broadly cover periodontal disease and tooth resorption, which affect more than 60 % of the cats that we see in our practice. Moreover, we have included new body condition and muscle mass charts. In short, this update makes the second edition of this Atlas an essential tool in daily veterinary practice.

I hope it helps you as much as it has helped me.

María Luisa Palmero
Director of the Gattos Hospital
AVEPA-accredited in Feline Medicine
Specialist in Endoscopy and Minimally Invasive Surgery (SpecEaMIS)

Table of contents

01 ANATOMY AND PHYSIOLOGY

02 MAIN CONDITIONS BY SYSTEM

1 Skeleton of the cat

Fibrous, cartilaginous and synovial joints

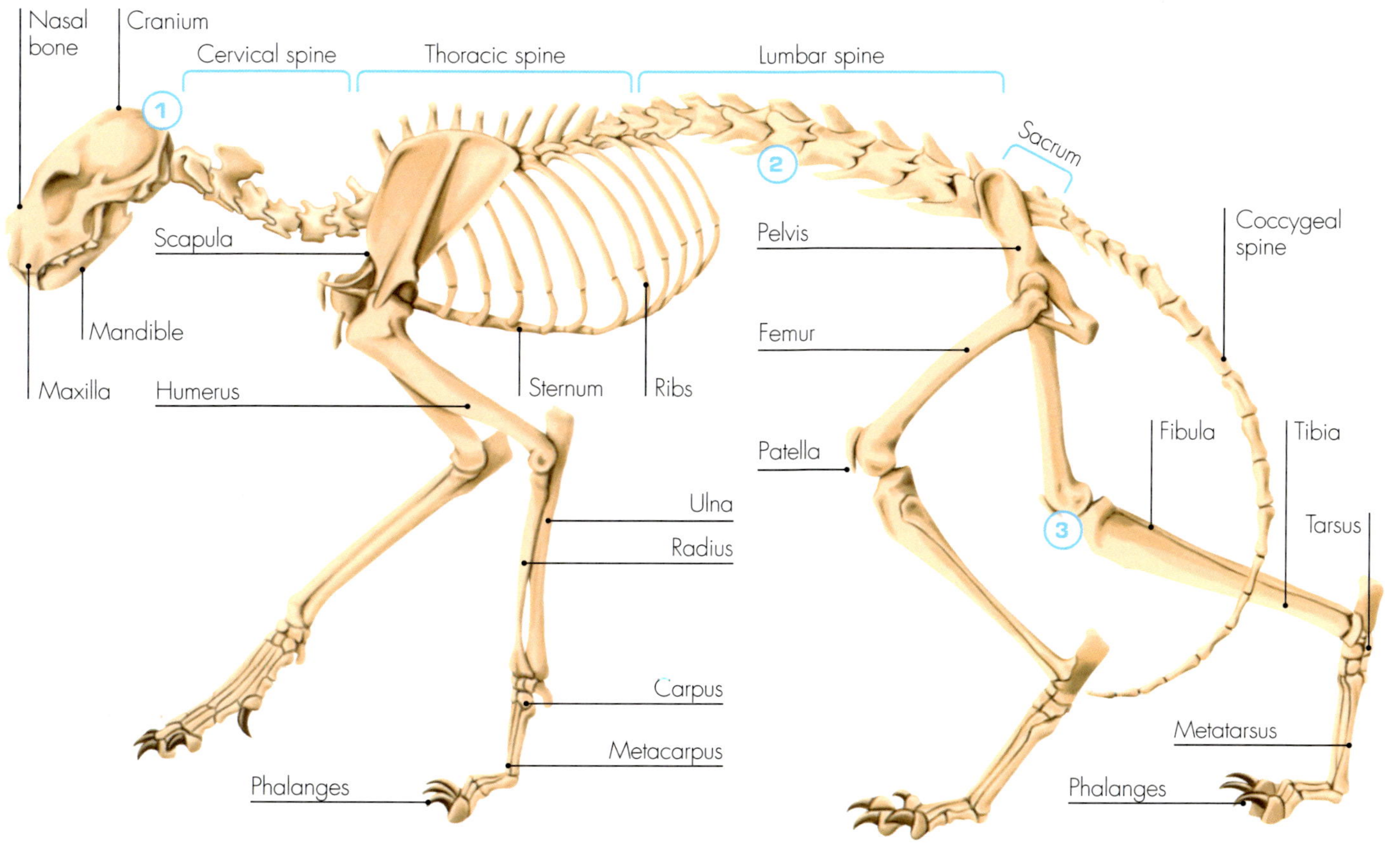

1 FIBROUS JOINT (cranial sutures)

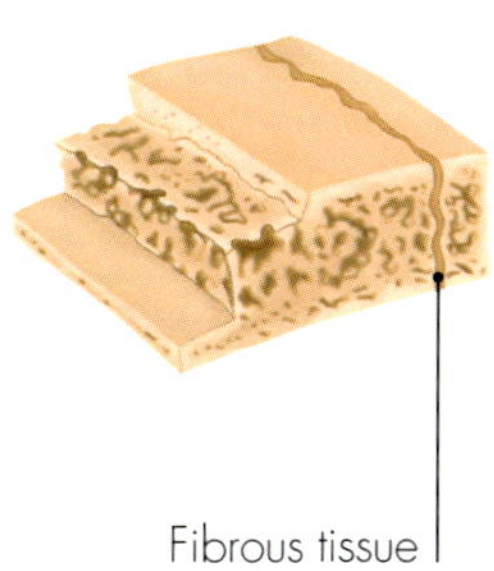

2 CARTILAGINOUS JOINT (intervertebral joints)

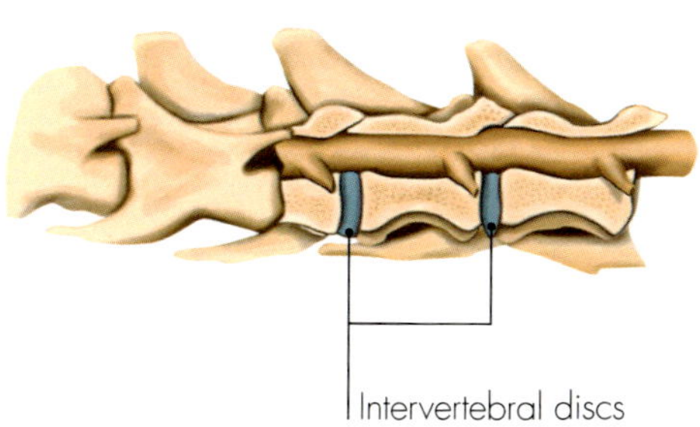

3 SYNOVIAL JOINT (stifle, elbow, shoulder, hip, etc.)

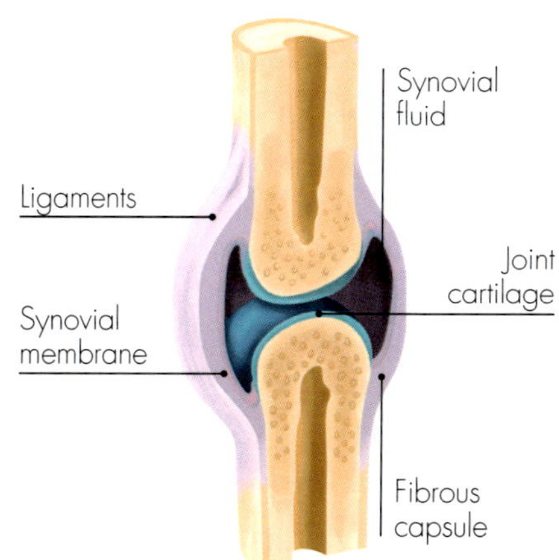

2 Muscles of the cat

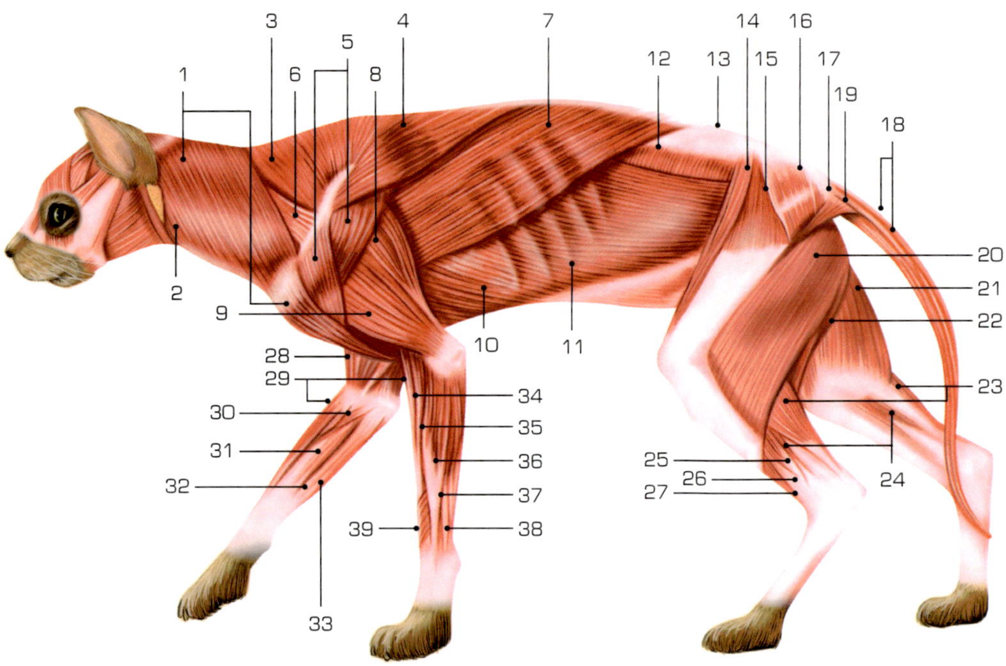

1. Brachiocephalic muscle (cleidocephalicus and cleidobrachialis)
2. Sternocephalic muscle
3. Trapezius muscle (cervical part)
4. Trapezius muscle (thoracic part)
5. Deltoid muscle
6. Omotransversarius muscle
7. Latissimus dorsi muscle
8. Triceps brachii muscle (long head)
9. Triceps brachii muscle (lateral head)
10. Deep pectoral muscle
11. Abdominal external oblique muscle
12. Abdominal internal oblique muscle
13. Thoracolumbar fascia
14. Sartorius muscle
15. Tensor fasciae latae muscle
16. Gluteus medius muscle
17. Gluteus superficialis muscle
18. Sacrocaudal muscles
19. Caudofemoralis muscles
20. Biceps femoris muscle
21. Semimembranosus muscle
22. Semitendinosus muscle
23. Gastrocnemius muscle
24. Deep digital flexor muscle
25. Lateral digital extensor muscle
26. Peroneus longus muscle
27. Tibialis cranialis muscle
28. Biceps brachii muscle
29. Brachioradialis muscle
30. Pronator teres muscle
31. Extensor carpi radialis muscle
32. Flexor carpi radialis muscle
33. Superficial digital flexor muscle
34. Extensor carpi radialis muscle
35. Extensor digitorum communis muscle
36. Extensor digitorum lateralis muscle
37. Extensor carpi ulnaris muscle
38. Flexor carpi ulnaris muscle
39. Digital abductor muscle

Muscles of the face

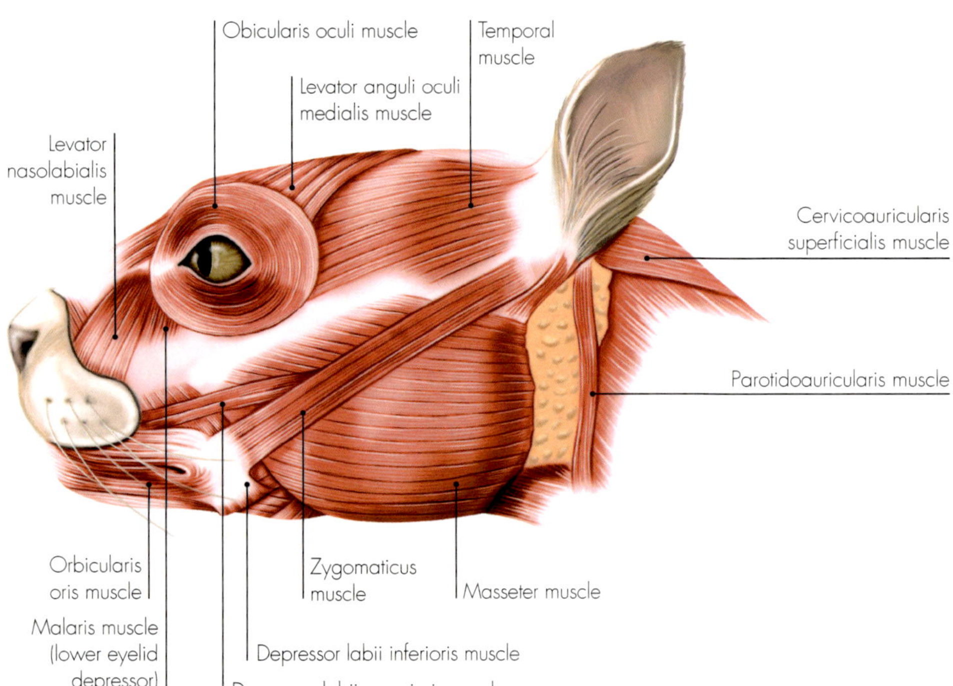

3 Abdominal organs of the cat

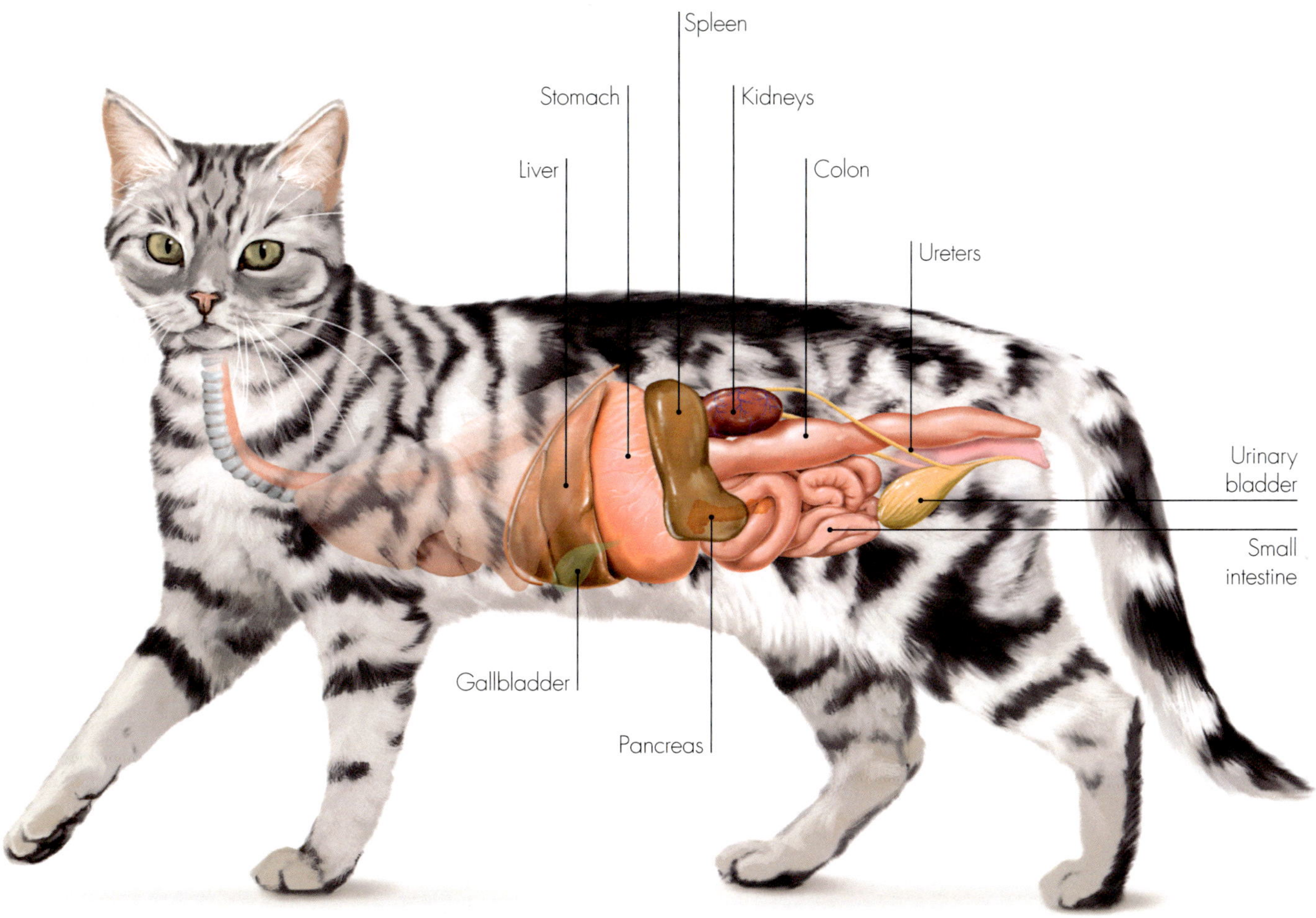

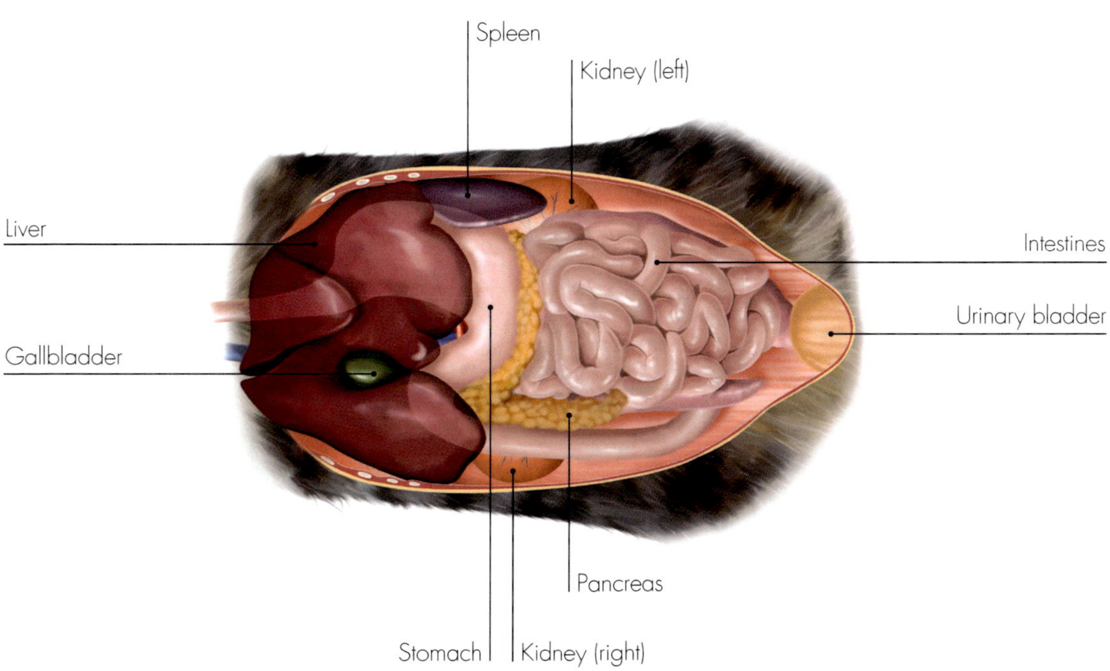

4 Cardiorespiratory system

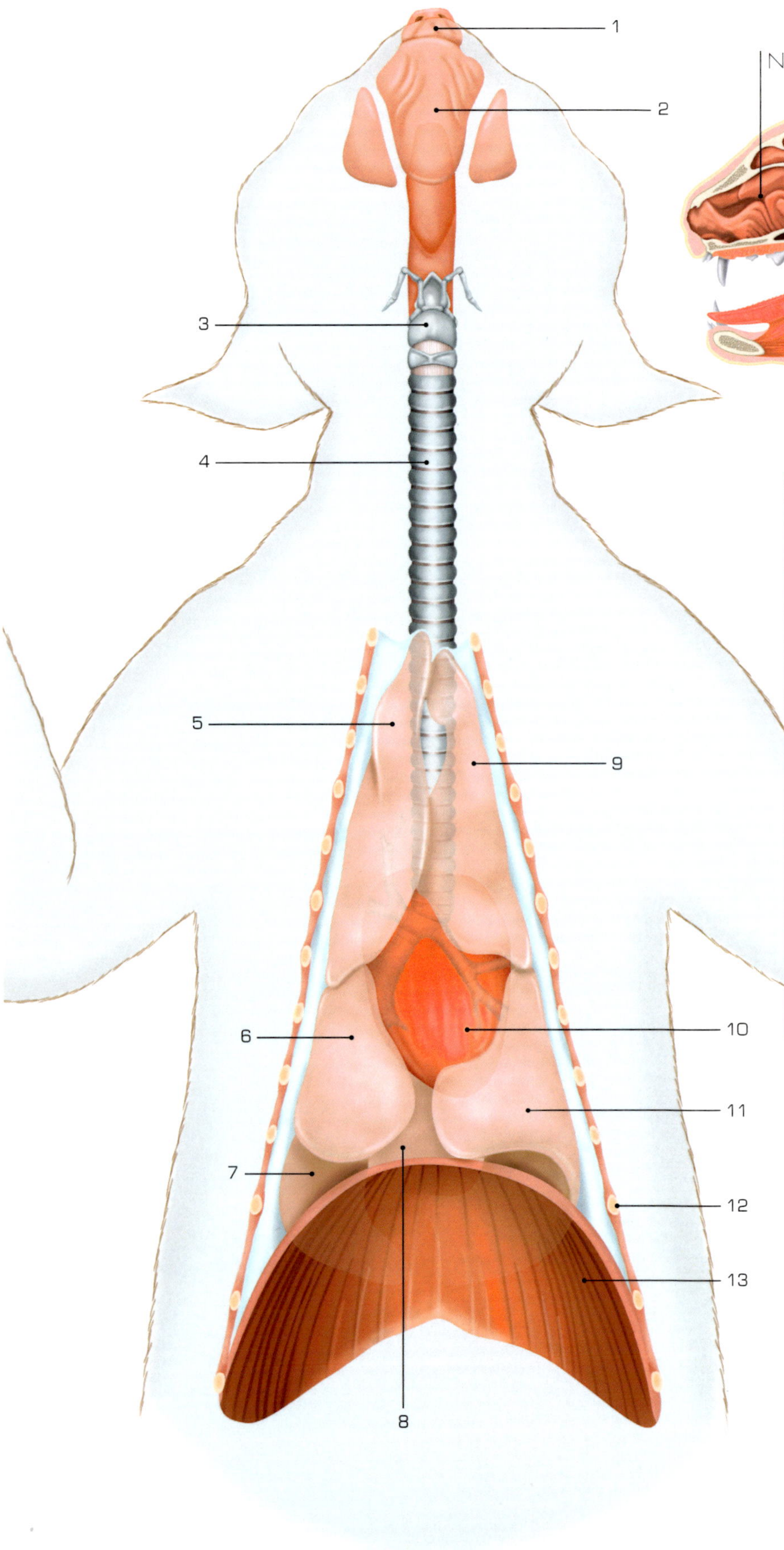

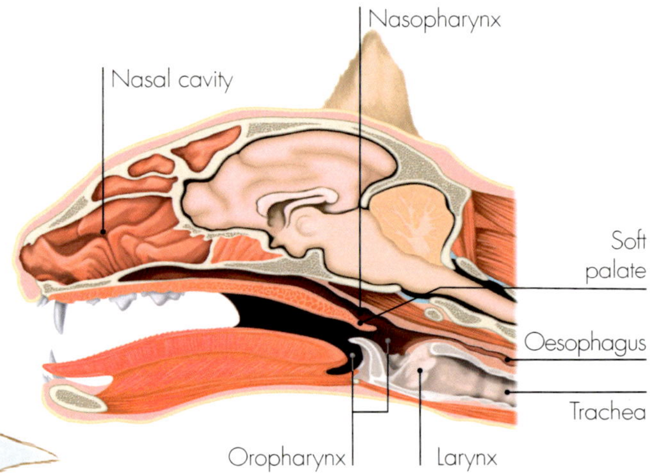

BLOOD CIRCULATION

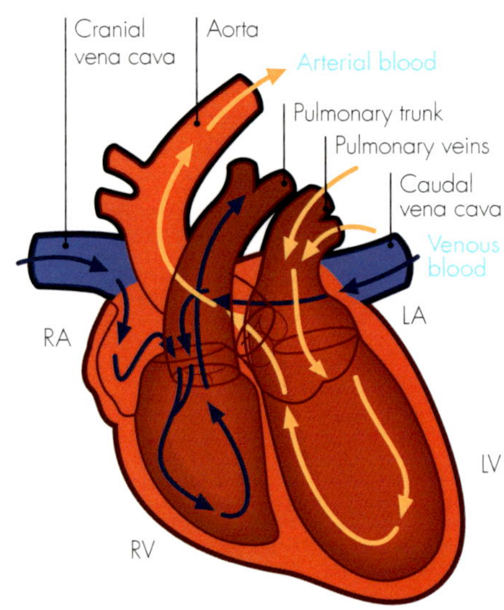

1. Nose
2. Nasal cavity
3. Larynx
4. Trachea
5. Right lung, cranial lobe
6. Right lung, middle lobe
7. Right lung, caudal lobe
8. Right lung, accessory lobe
9. Left lung, cranial lobe
10. Heart
11. Left lung, caudal lobe
12. Ribs
13. Diaphragm

GUIDELINES

5 Body condition and muscle mass index

Body condition

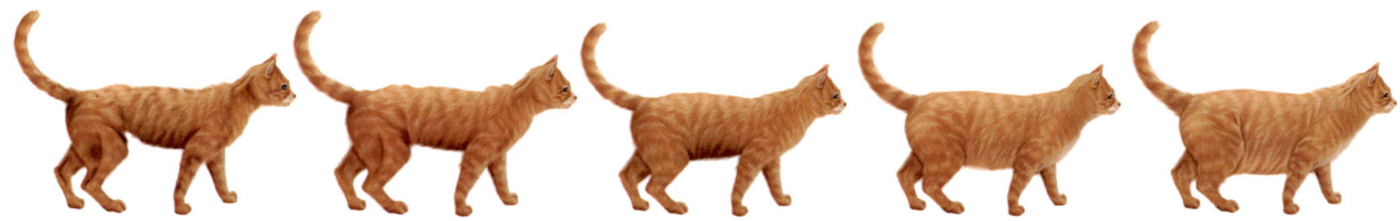

1, 2 Extremely thin	3, 4 Thin	5 Optimal	6, 7 Overweight	8, 9 Obese
■ Ribs are visible. ■ Absence of abdominal fat. ■ Vertebrae are visible.	■ Ribs are very easily palpable. ■ Absence of abdominal fat. ■ Vertebrae easily palpated.	■ Well proportioned with adequate abdominal fat. ■ Linear silhouette, abdomen does not protrude.	■ Ribs not easily palpable. ■ Obvious abdominal fat. ■ Vertebrae palpated with difficulty. ■ Rounded silhouette.	■ Ribs not palpable. ■ Abundant abdominal fat. ■ Vertebrae barely palpable. ■ Very rounded silhouette.

Muscle mass index

- The same cat can be overweight and also have a reduced muscle mass due to osteoarthritis and dietary deficiencies, or can have a reduced body condition but good muscle mass owing to high physical activity. Therefore, it is important to evaluate both factors.
- Sarcopaenia (generalised reduction in muscle mass) causes weakness.
- A loss of muscle mass in a muscle group indicates joint disease.
- Treatment includes dietary changes, analgesia, and rehabilitation.

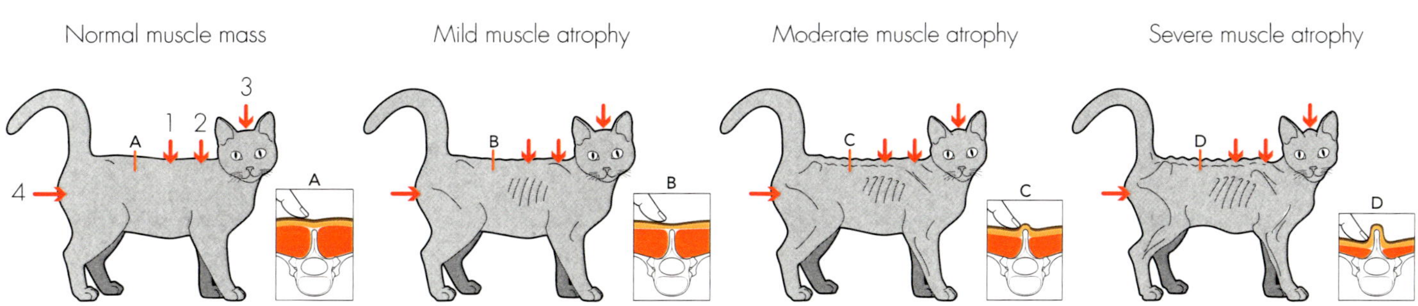

Where to palpate:

1. Spinal column
2. Scapulae
3. Skull
4. Ischial tuberosity

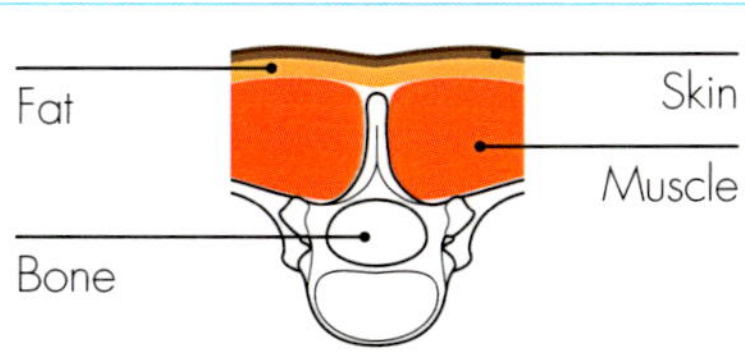

Based on the "Muscle Condition Score" (WSAVA) developed by Tufts University, 2013.

GUIDELINES

6 Pain scale according to facial expression (grimace scale)

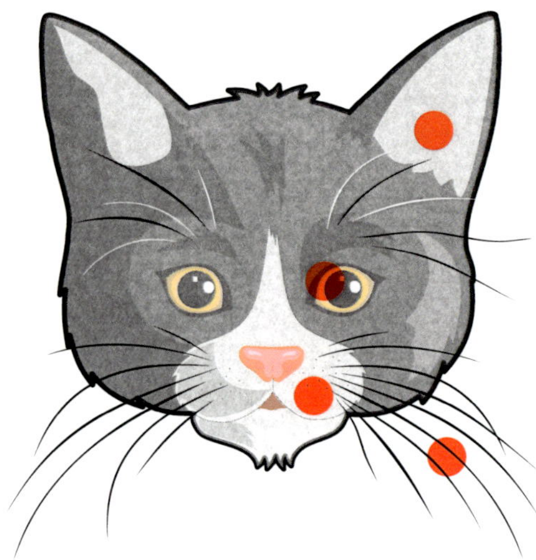

This scale enables recognition of **acute pain** in cats, including those that have been sedated with acepromazine/buprenorphine and are recovering from anaesthesia. It is based on a study conducted in 2020 (Clinical applicability of the Feline Grimace Scale).

0 = absent	1 = moderately present	2 = markedly present
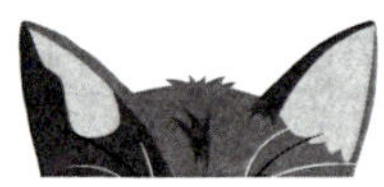 Ears forward	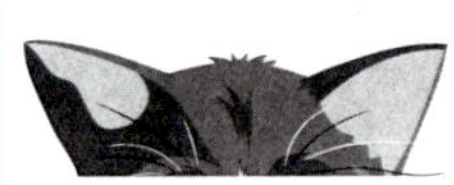 Ears slightly pulled apart	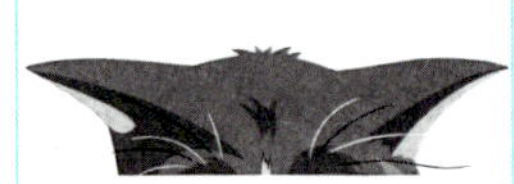 Ears flattened
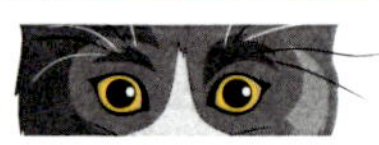 Rounded eyes	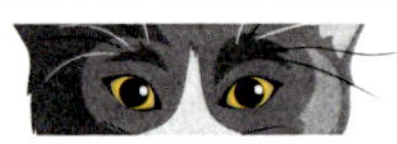 Eyes slightly closed	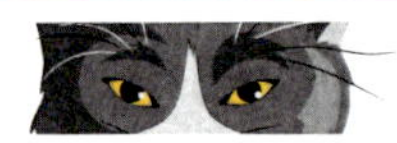 Squinting eyes
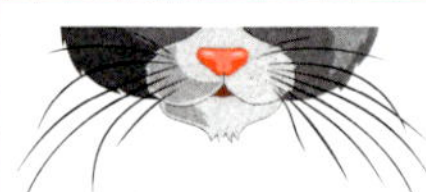 Whiskers curved downwards	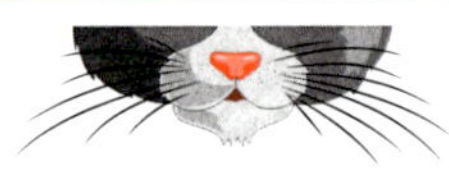 Whiskers straight or curved upwards	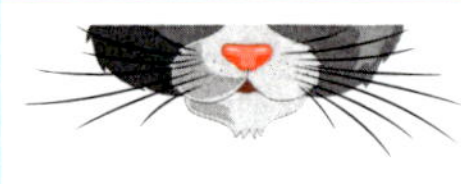 Whiskers straight and separated
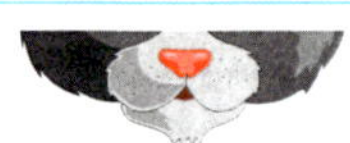 Relaxed muzzle (round)	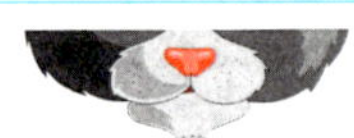 Muzzle slightly tense	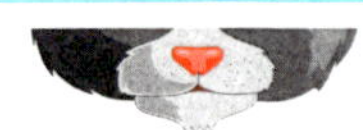 Tense muzzle (elliptical)

How to use the scale

Four sites on the face are evaluated: the ears, eyes, whiskers, and cheeks. Each site on the face is scored 0, 1, or 2, and the total score is summed:

- Score <4: indicative of no pain.
- Score ≥4: immediate analgesia required.
- Score of 8: intense pain.

The cat should be reassessed to verify the efficacy of the analgesia used.

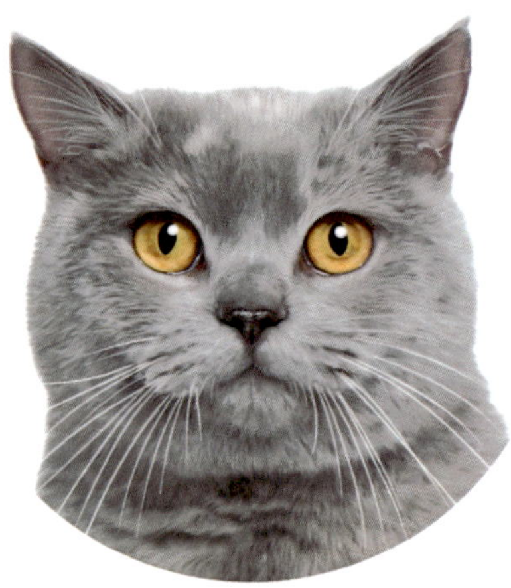

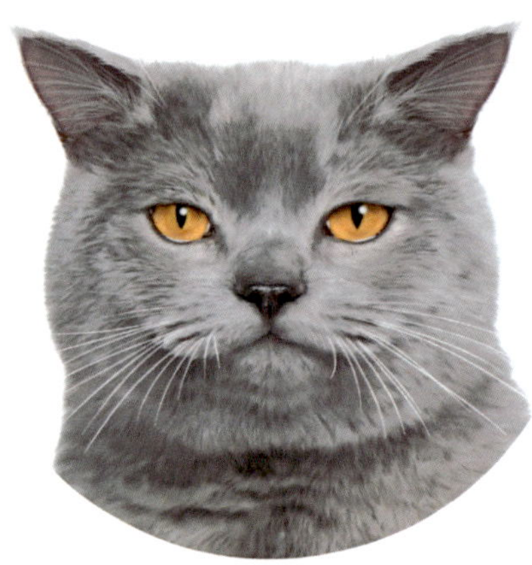

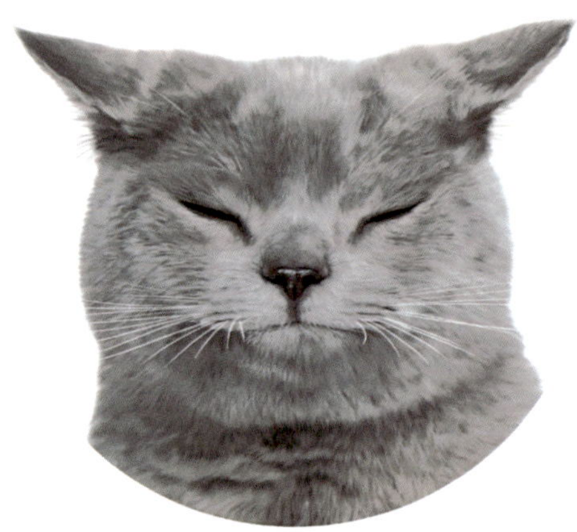

Score of 0 (no pain):

- Ears forward.
- Rounded eyes.
- Relaxed muzzle (round).
- Whiskers curved downwards.

Score of 1 (moderate pain):

- Ears slightly pulled apart.
- Eyes somewhat closed.
- Muzzle slightly tense.
- Whiskers straight or curved upwards.

Score of 2 (severe pain):

- Ears flattened.
- Squinting eyes.
- Tense muzzle (elliptical).
- Whiskers straight and separated.

MUSCULOSKELETAL SYSTEM

7 Osteoarthritis

Degenerative joint disease

Osteoarthritis may go unnoticed as its symptoms are attributed to age instead of joint pain. The most affected joints are the hip and the elbows, and osteoarthritis is very commonly observed in several joints in the same cat.

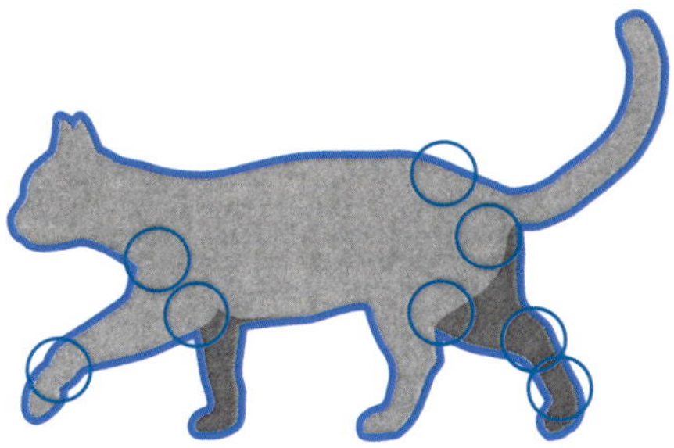

90 % of cats over 12 years of age show signs of joint degeneration.

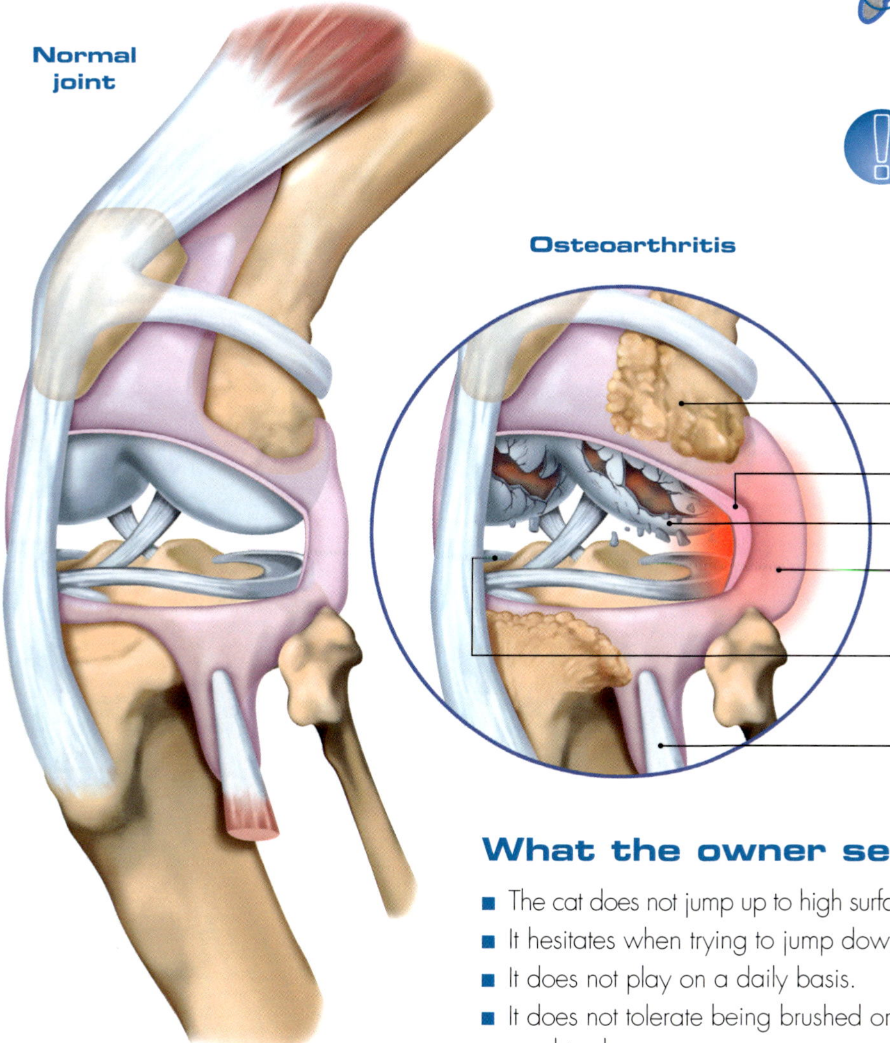

What the owner sees

- The cat does not jump up to high surfaces, or uses intermediate steps to do so.
- It hesitates when trying to jump down.
- It does not play on a daily basis.
- It does not tolerate being brushed or being held in someone's arms, when it used to do so.
- More frequent meowing.
- Decreased grooming.

Medical treatment

- Multimodal analgesic therapy.
- Rehabilitation.
- Anti-NGF (nerve growth factor) monoclonal antibody therapy.

Dietary treatment

Dietary modification, with diets rich in glycosaminoglycans and essential fatty acids.

Recommendations

- Prevention of obesity.
- Environmental modifications to facilitate mobility and access to the animal's favourite places.

MUSCULOSKELETAL SYSTEM

8 How to detect pain

Cats show changes in behaviour rather than lameness in response to joint pain. A recent study found that asking the following questions during the consultation was effective in detecting osteoarthrosis with a sensitivity of 99 % and a specificity of 100 % (Enomoto *et al.*, Development of a checklist for the detection of degenerative joint disease-associated pain in cats. *J Feline Med Surg*, 2020).

Does your cat jump up normally?

If the cat hesitates before jumping up to a spot that previously caused it no trouble, it is a sign of pain.

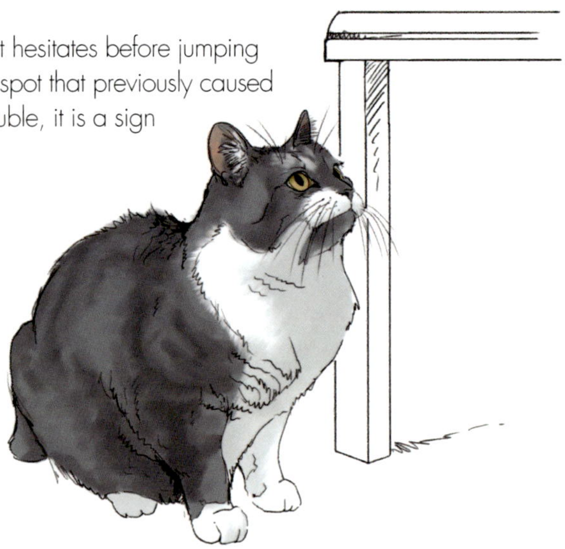

Does your cat jump down normally?

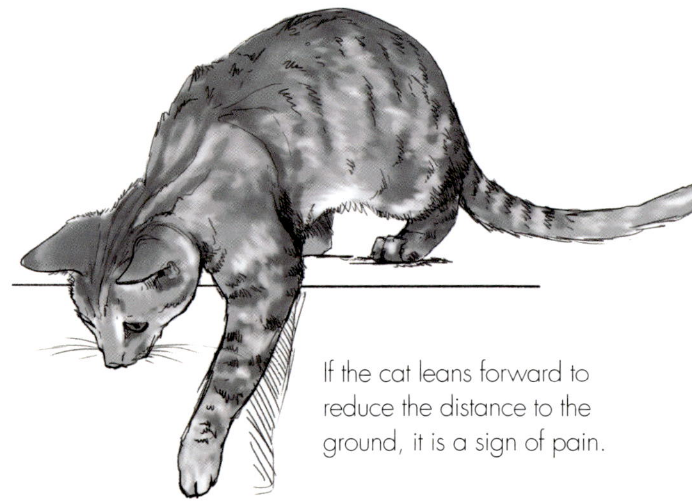

If the cat leans forward to reduce the distance to the ground, it is a sign of pain.

Does your cat run normally?

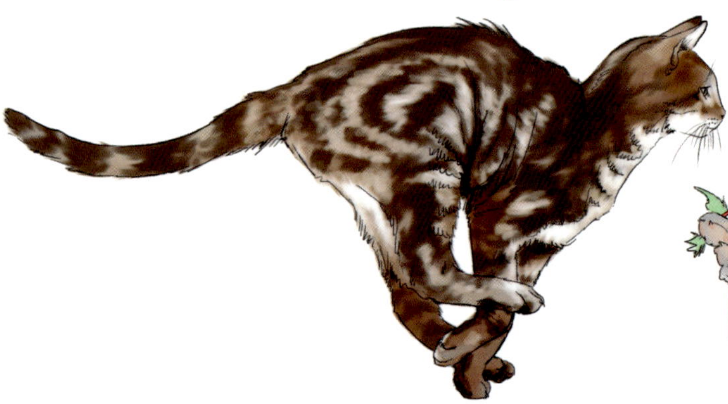

Does your cat climb up or down stairs or steps normally?

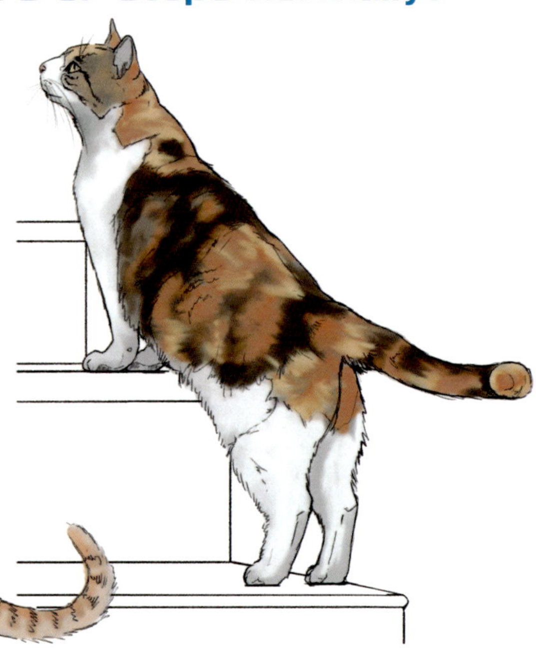

Does your cat play with objects normally?

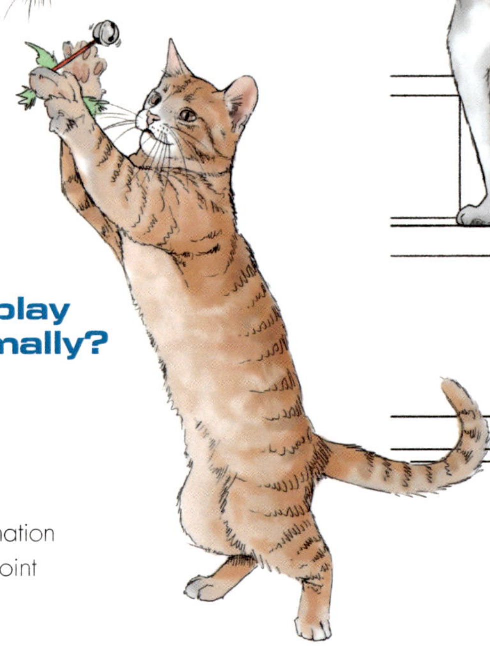

Interpretation of responses

If any of the questions receives a NO, a joint examination and radiographs should be performed to locate the joint affected by osteoarthrosis.

MUSCULOSKELETAL SYSTEM

9 Hip dysplasia

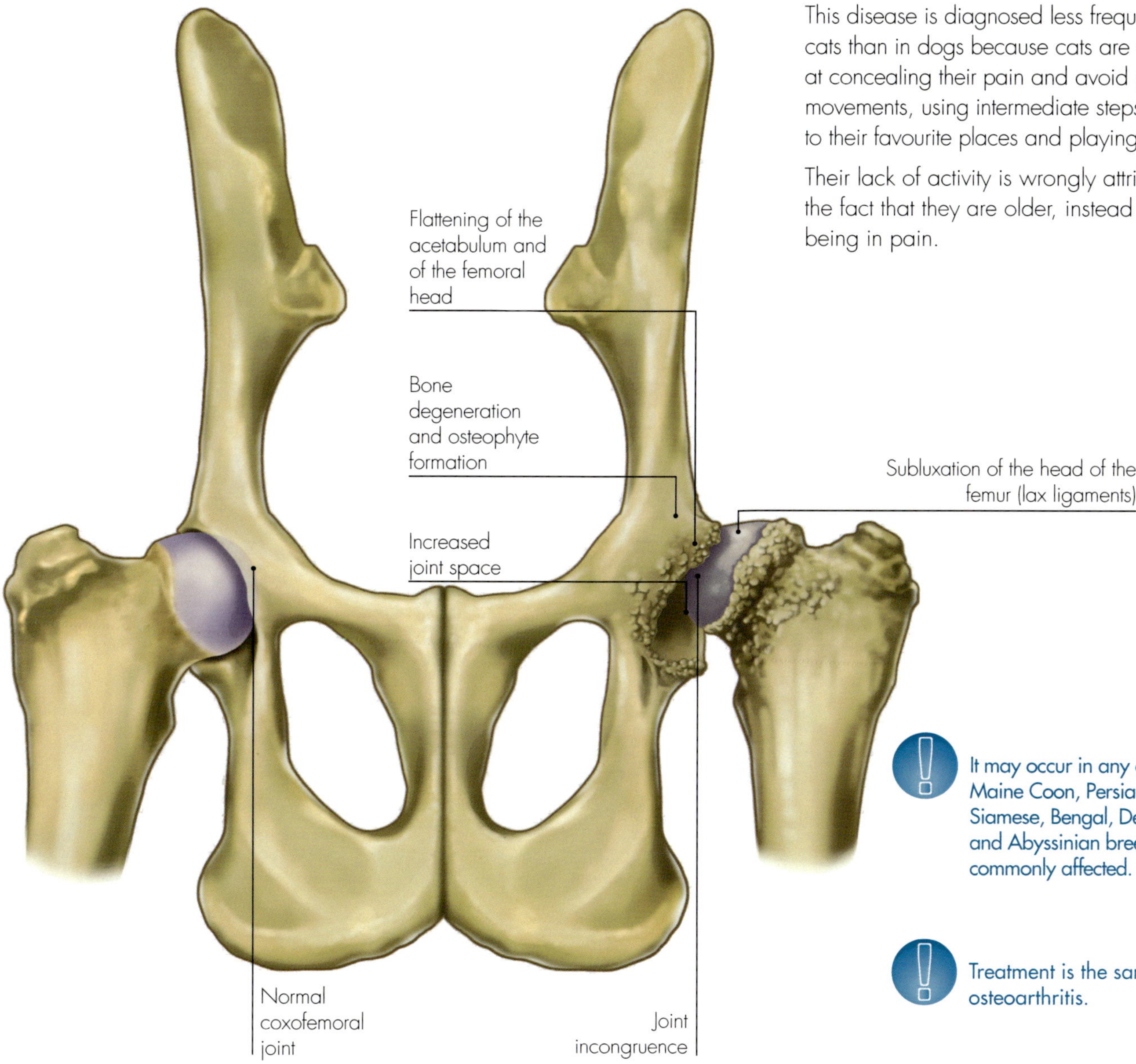

This disease is diagnosed less frequently in cats than in dogs because cats are very good at concealing their pain and avoid painful movements, using intermediate steps to jump up to their favourite places and playing less.

Their lack of activity is wrongly attributed to the fact that they are older, instead of to them being in pain.

It may occur in any cat, but the Maine Coon, Persian, Himalayan, Siamese, Bengal, Devon Rex and Abyssinian breeds are most commonly affected.

Treatment is the same as for osteoarthritis.

Clinical signs

In cats suffering from joint degeneration and osteoarthritis, we will observe:

- Stiffness of hind limbs when walking.
- Clumsier movements when jumping up to their favourite places or they may not reach high places in one jump.
- Lameness, although it is uncommon.
- Their daily play sessions are reduced.
- They may become more irritable when their hind limbs are touched.

MUSCULOSKELETAL SYSTEM

10 Sacrococcygeal luxation

Usual causes

- Abrupt pulling of the tail.
- Road traffic accidents.
- Dog bites.
- Other traumas (e.g. gunshots).

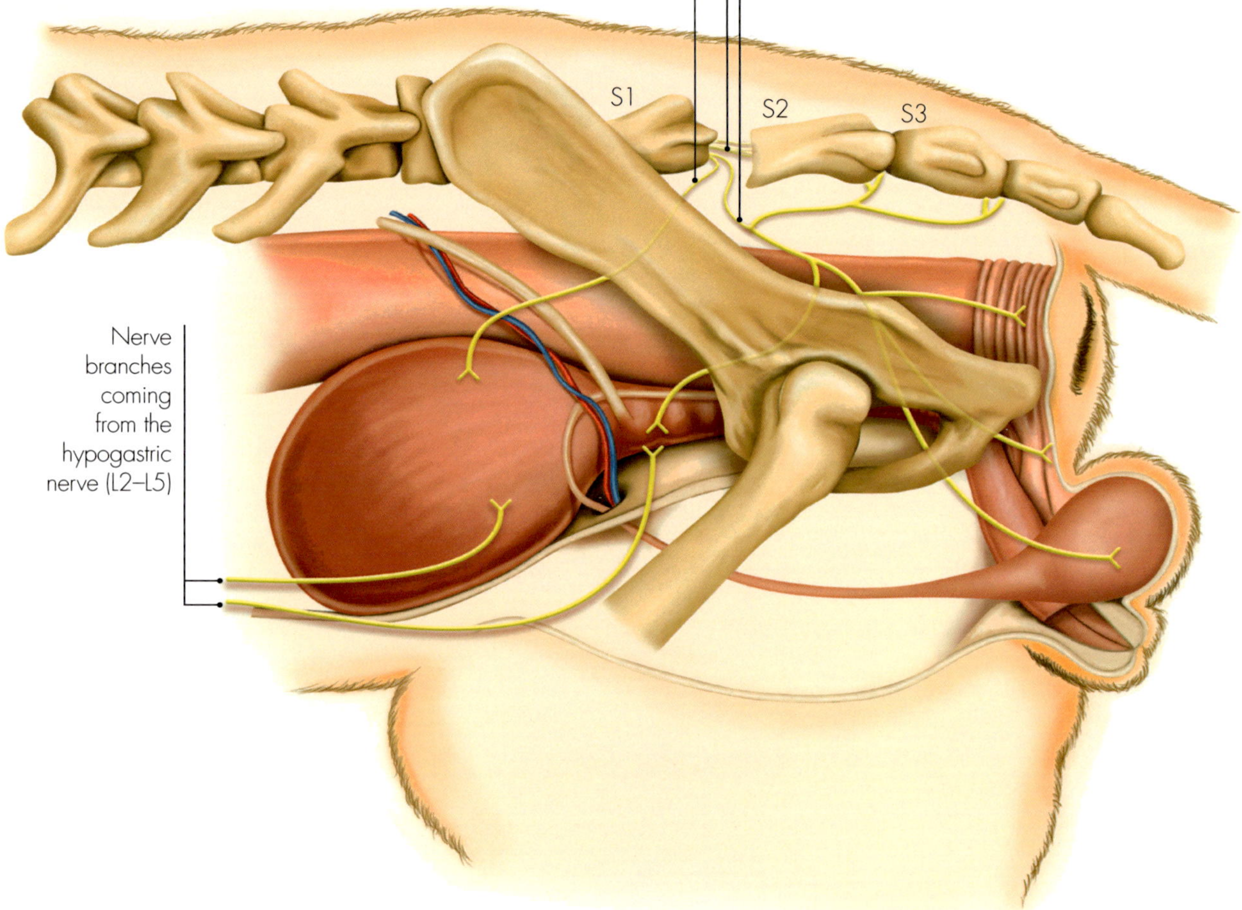

Clinical signs

- Problems of micturition (incontinence) and defecation and loss of perineal sensitivity due to:
  - Lesion of the pudendal nerve: sensory and motor innervation of the anal and urethral sphincters, and sensitivity of the perineum and genital organs.
  - Lesion of the pelvic nerves: innervation of the rectum, genitalia and detrusor muscle of the bladder. Urinary incontinence.
- Flaccidity or paralysis of the tail due to a lesion of the caudal nerves (sensory and motor innervations).
- Mild or moderate alterations in the hind limbs due to a secondary involvement of the sciatic nerve.

RENAL AND URINARY SYSTEM

11 Chronic kidney disease (CKD)

It is one of the most common conditions in feline medicine. It affects animals at any age, but the probability of suffering from it doubles from 7-10 years of age. Cats do not show clinical signs until at least 70 % of the functional nephrons have been lost.

Accurate diagnosis and control of disease progression require blood and urine tests, urine culture, measurement of protein:creatinine ratio, evaluation of blood pressure, abdominal ultrasound, and radiology.

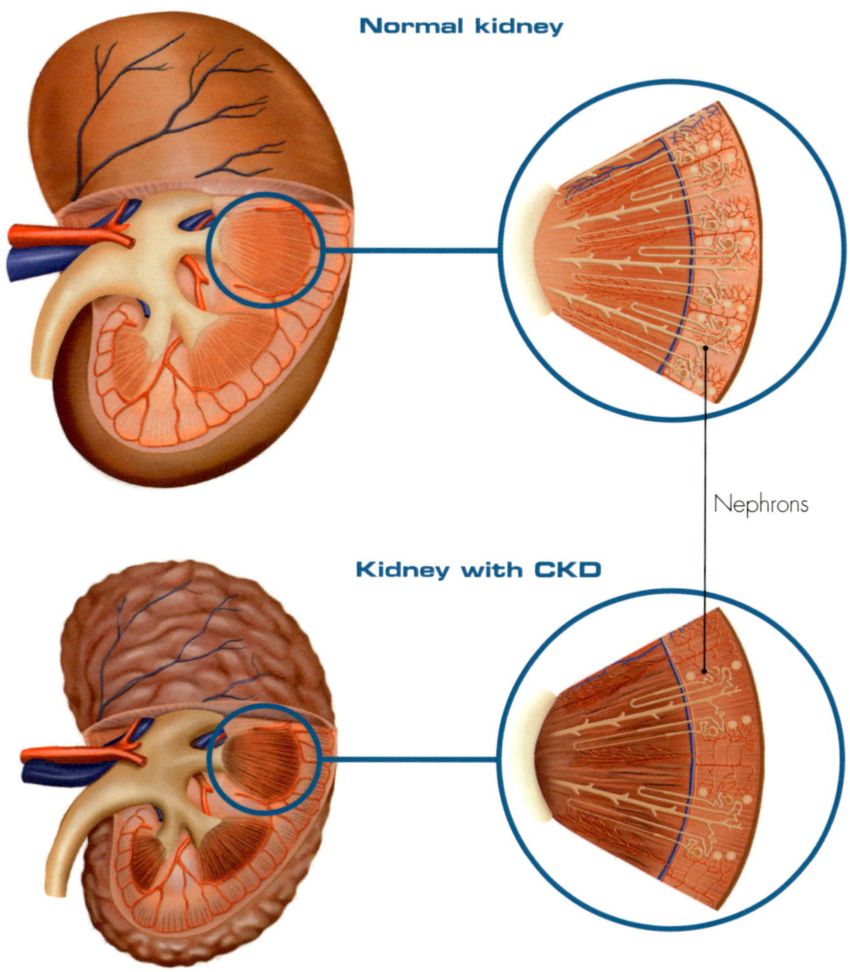

Progression of CKD

1. Kidney damage
2. Reduction of the number and function of nephrons
3. Progressive reduction of glomerular filtration
4. Increased levels of urea and creatinine and other products excreted by the kidneys
5. Onset of clinical signs: polyuria/polydipsia, progressive loss of weight, chronic vomiting, loss of appetite
6. If it progresses, it may lead to death

Grade	Serum creatinine
I	<1.6 mg/dl
II	1.6-2.8 mg/dl
III	2.9-5 mg/dl
IV	>5.0 mg/dl

IRIS (International Renal Interest Society) Guidelines 2016, revised in 2019.

Causes of CKD

Congenital:

- Renal aplasia, dysplasia and hypoplasia.
- Renal amyloidosis.
- Feline polycystic kidney disease.

Acquired:

- Idiopathic tubulo-interstitial nephritis.
- Pyelonephritis.
- Glomerulonephritis.
- Acquired amyloidosis.
- Nephrotoxins.
- Hypercalcaemia.
- Hydronephrosis (chronic ureteral obstruction).
- Renal lymphoma.
- Progression of acute kidney disease.
- Feline infectious peritonitis.

RENAL AND URINARY SYSTEM

12 Acute renal failure (ARF)

Acute renal failure (ARF) describes the acute collapse of renal function with a decrease in glomerular filtration rate, which leads to the development of azotaemia, electrolyte disturbances, and acid–base disturbances.

Causes

- Prerenal ARF: ischaemia (dehydration, hypovolaemia, sepsis, heart failure, hypotension) or drugs that alter perfusion (NSAIDs and ACEIs).
- Renal ARF: tubular necrosis (ischaemia, toxins), pyelonephritis, glomerulonephritis, vasculitis, systemic disease (FIP, neoplasia, sepsis), or untreated prerenal ARF.
- Postrenal ARF: ureteral or urethral obstruction, bladder or ureteral rupture.

Normal kidney

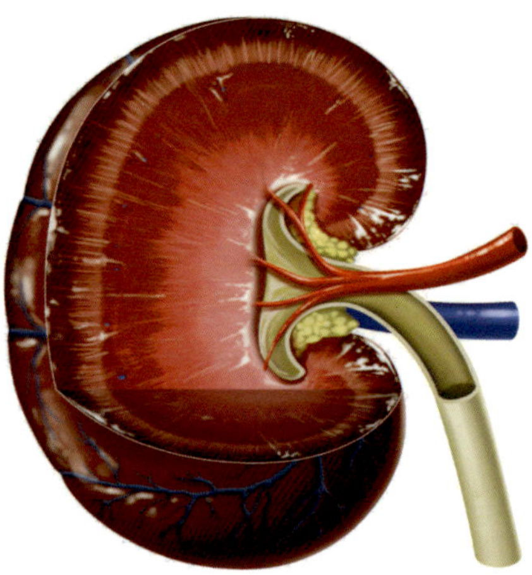

The prognosis is reserved, with a mortality rate of up to 55 %.

Acute renal failure

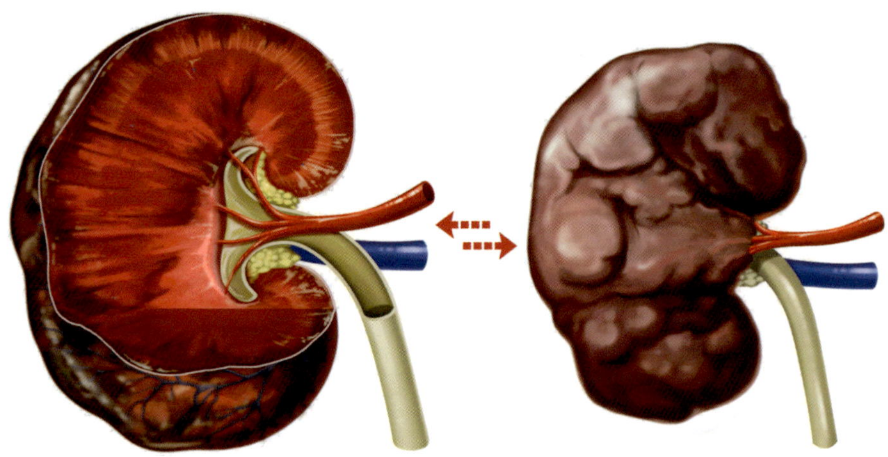

Normal or enlarged kidneys are a classic sign of ARF

Small kidneys are indicative of acute-on-chronic renal failure

- Frequently the development of ARF leads to chronic kidney disease (CKD), as kidney function cannot fully recover.
- Cats with CKD frequently develop ARF due to changes in perfusion (dehydration) or infections (pyelonephritis). This process is known as **acute-on-chronic renal failure**.

Diagnosis

- Blood test: variable azotaemia and hyperkalaemia.
- Urinalysis with urine protein:creatinine ratio (UPC) and culture.
- Abdominal ultrasound and radiography: ESSENTIAL for diagnosis.

The factors associated with higher mortality are hyperkalaemia and oliguria.

Grade	Clinical presentation	Serum creatinine
ARF I	Without azotaemia	<1.6 mg/dl
ARF II	Mild	1.7–2.5 mg/dl
ARF III	Moderate	2.6–5 mg/dl
ARF IV	Severe	5.1–10 mg/dl
ARF V	Severe	>10 mg/dl

IRIS (International Renal Interest Society) Guidelines 2016, revised in 2019.

RENAL AND URINARY SYSTEM

13 Pyelonephritis

Pyelonephritis is a common cause of acute kidney disease and exacerbation of chronic kidney disease. Bacterial infection reaches the kidney either ascending from the bladder or via the bloodstream.

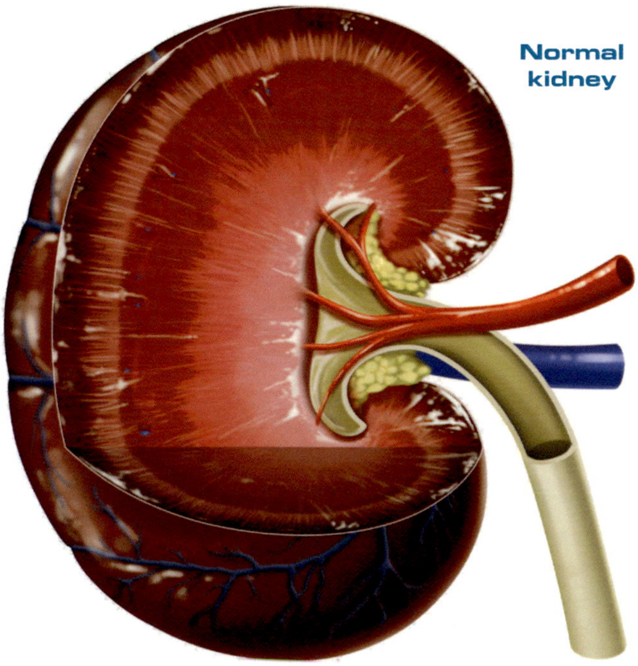

Clinical signs

- Acute depression.
- Kidney pain (can be difficult to detect).
- Lower urinary tract signs (inadequate urination and dysuria): may be present if there is associated bacterial cystitis.
- Fever (rare).

Diagnosis

- Urine culture.
- Ultrasound-guided puncture of the renal pelvis and culture when possible.

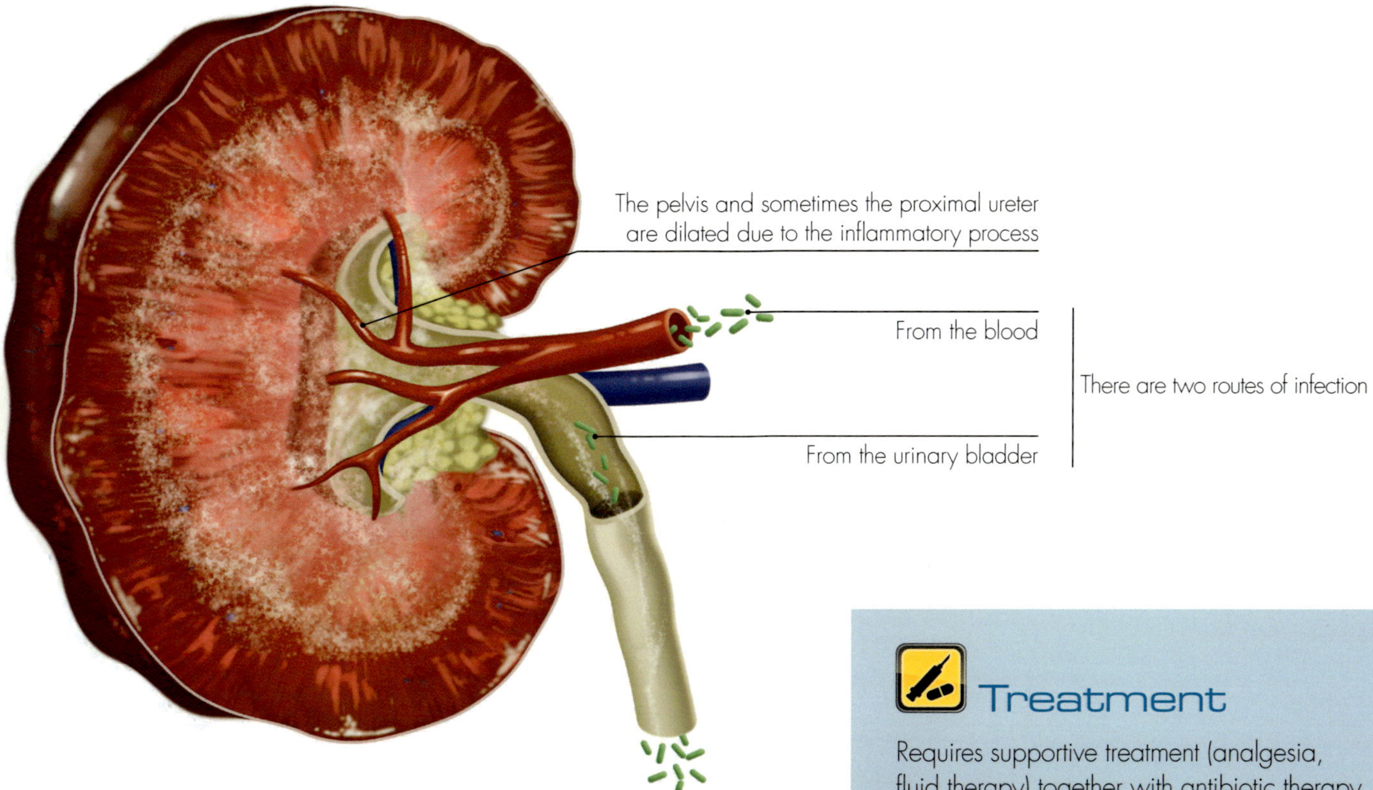

Treatment

Requires supportive treatment (analgesia, fluid therapy) together with antibiotic therapy for 14 days.

RENAL AND URINARY SYSTEM

14 Lilium poisoning

Ingestion of plants of the genera *Lilium* and *Hemerocallis* (lilies and daylilies) is associated with the development of ARF. These plants contain an as-yet-unidentified toxin that causes tubular necrosis. Even a small amount can be fatal.

Any part of the plant is toxic: flower, stem, leaves, pollen. The flower is the most toxic part.

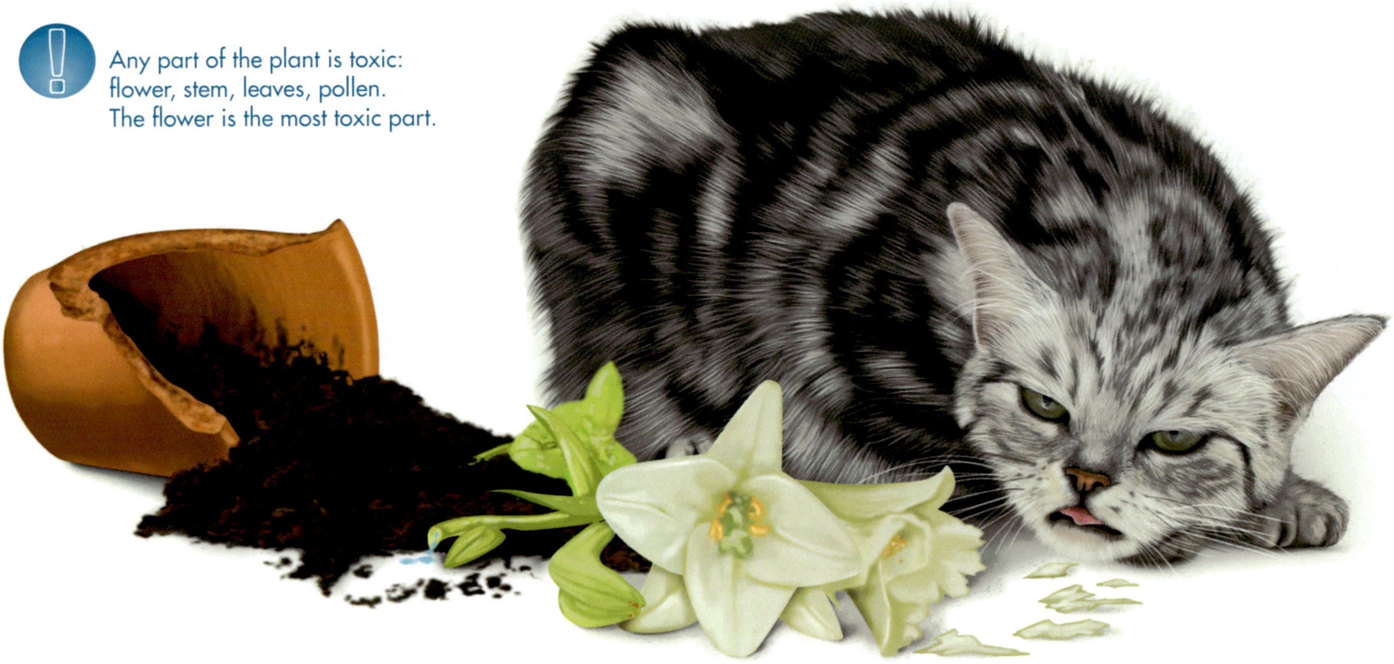

Clinical signs

- After ingestion of the plant, clinical signs of acute renal failure appear within 12–36 hours.
- Acute vomiting may be observed, followed by depression, anorexia, and hypersalivation.
- Oliguria/anuria can occur.
- Depending on the amount ingested, affected cats can die within 3–5 days.

Course

Cats that survive develop chronic kidney disease of varying degrees of severity.

Treatment

- In the event that the cat has been exposed to the toxin recently and has not vomited, induce vomiting, perform gastric lavage, or use activated charcoal.
- If hours have passed since ingestion, the cat should be hospitalised to maintain hydration and treat symptomatically.
- There is no specific treatment for the toxin.

RENAL AND URINARY SYSTEM

15 Systemic hypertension (SH)

It is the sustained increase in arterial pressure (AP) above values considered as normal. Values of systolic AP > 140 mmHg obtained with an HDO device (high-definition oscillometry) and > 160 mmHg obtained with a Doppler ultrasound device are indicative of hypertension.

Blood pressure should be taken at least 10 minutes after the animal has entered the consultation room. Five consecutive determinations must be carried out, after which the highest and lowest values are excluded and the mean calculated.

Causes

- Idiopathic or essential (the cause is unknown).
- Secondary to:
  - Kidney disease.
  - Hyperthyroidism.
  - After the treatment of hyperthyroidism (20 % of the cats treated).
  - Hyperaldosteronism.
  - Pheochromocytoma.
- White coat hypertension.

Consequences

- Hypertensive cats may be asymptomatic for months or years, until tissue damage is evident.
- Organs that suffer damage:
  - Heart.
  - Brain.
  - Kidney.
  - Eyes.

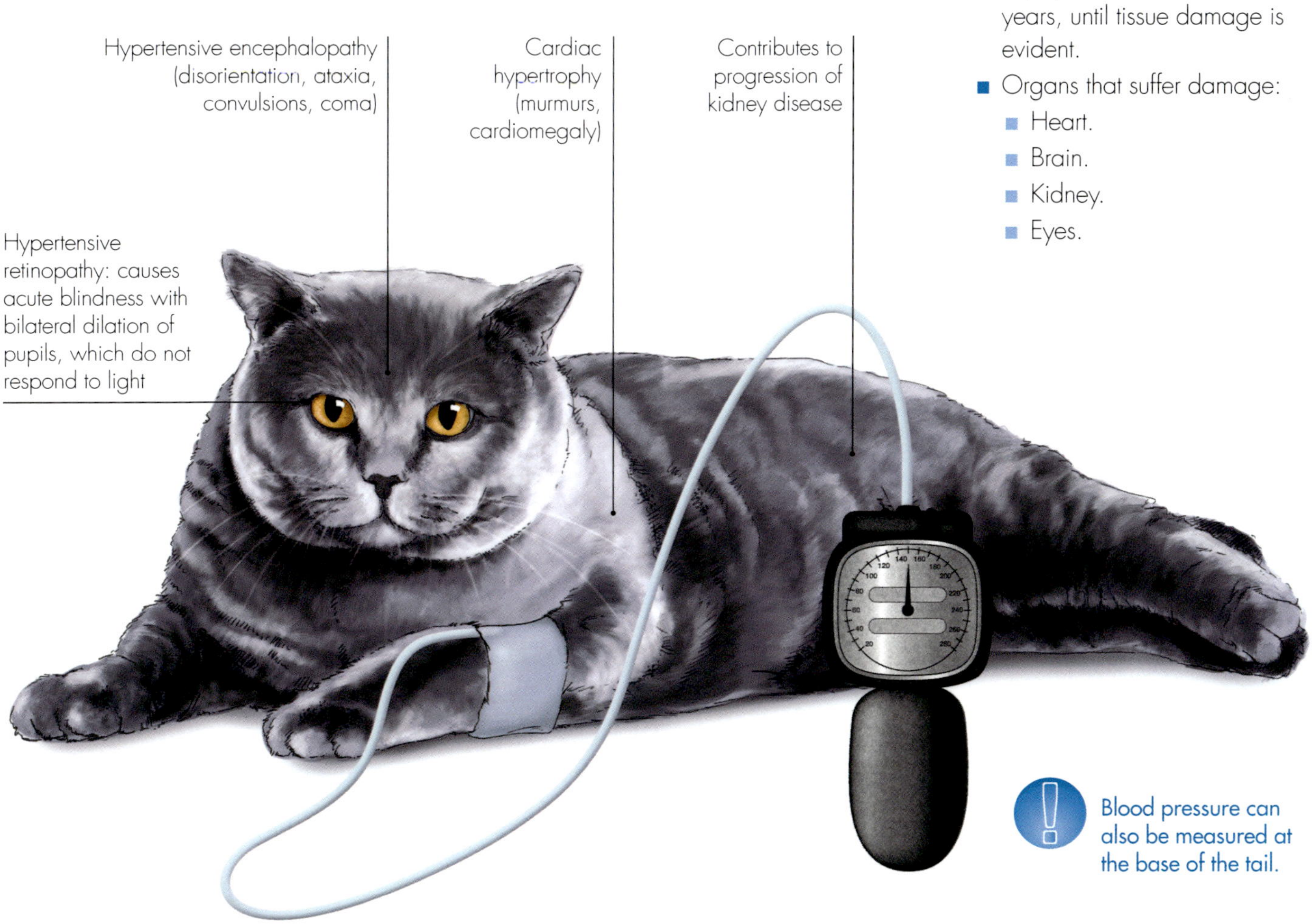

Blood pressure can also be measured at the base of the tail.

RENAL AND URINARY SYSTEM

16 Ureteral obstruction

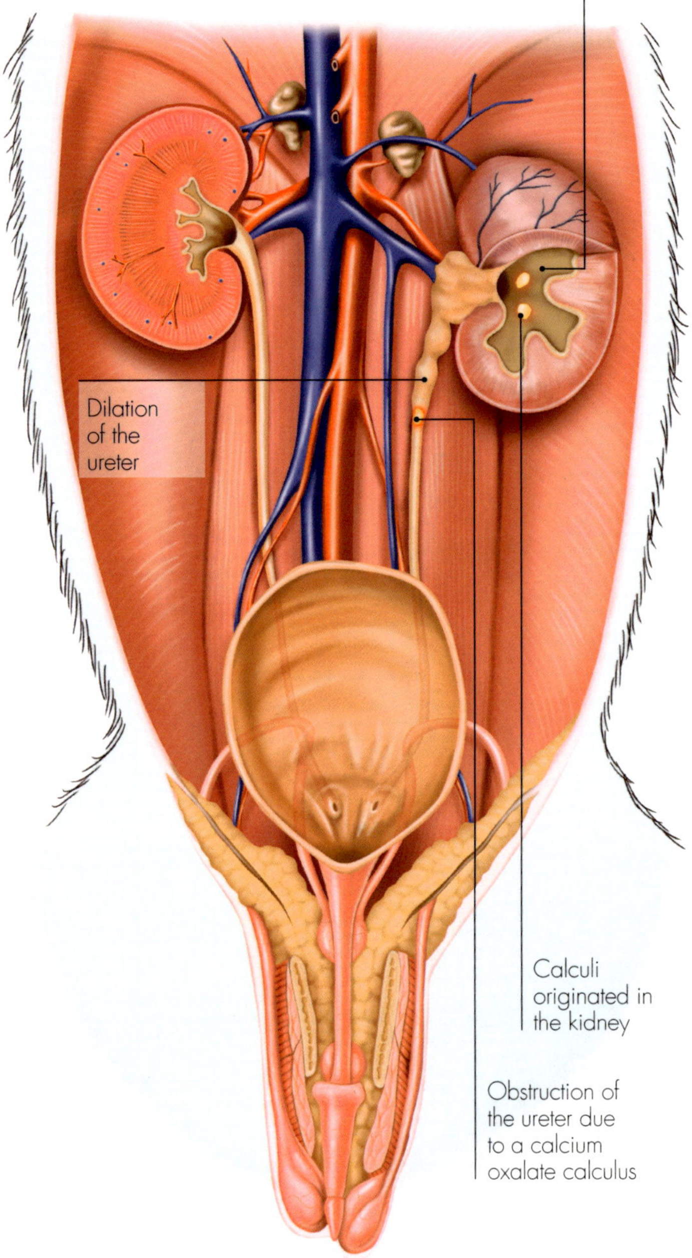

It is a frequent cause of chronic and acute kidney disease in cats of any age and sex. Bilateral ureteral obstruction is commonly observed.

Its diagnosis is made by means of abdominal radiographs and a high-definition ultrasound scan.

Causes

- Intraluminal:
  - Ureteroliths (80 %).
  - Clots.
  - Purulent aggregates (pyelonephritis).
- Intraparietal:
  - Congenital stenosis.
  - Secondary stenosis following ureteral surgery, inflammatory processes, passage of a calculus, infection, neoplasia, or granuloma.
- Extraparietal:
  - Retrocaval ureter (congenital).
  - Retroperitoneal fibrosis due to neoplasia or surgery.
  - Retroperitoneal masses.
  - Carcinoma of the bladder trigone.
  - Accidental ligation of ureters.

Medical treatment

- Intravenous fluid therapy for azotaemia.
- Smooth muscle relaxants to facilitate passage of the calculus.
- Analgesics.

Surgical treatment

- Ureterotomy.
- Subcutaneous ureteral bypass (SUB).
- Ureteral endoprosthesis (stent).

RENAL AND URINARY SYSTEM

17 Techniques for resolution of ureteral obstruction

Currently there are three techniques used to resolve ureteral obstruction: ureterotomy, endoprosthesis (stent), and subcutaneous bypass. All have their advantages and disadvantages.

Ureterotomy

- Using this technique, the ureter is dissected and the calculus is removed.
- This is performed if there a single obstruction located in the proximal third of the ureter.
- Advantages: definitive technique that avoids the persistence of materials that cause infections or migrations.
- Complications: leaks, stenosis, re-obstruction.

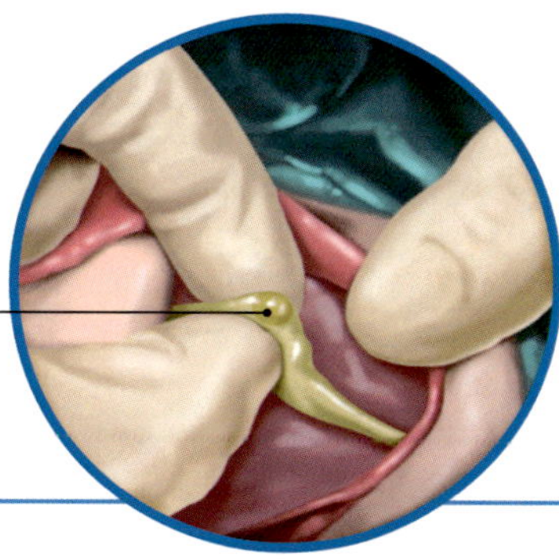

Endoprosthesis (stent)

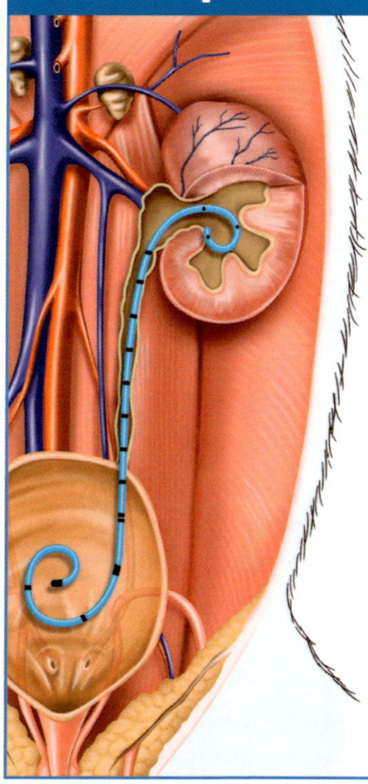

- Consists of placing a guide that passes through the ureter, from the bladder to the interior of the renal pelvis. This guide runs parallel to the calculi.
- This is achieved by open surgery or by endoscopy in females.
- Complications: ureteral rupture during the procedure, dysuria, haematuria, urinary infections, stent migration, calcification.

Subcutaneous ureteral bypass (SUB)

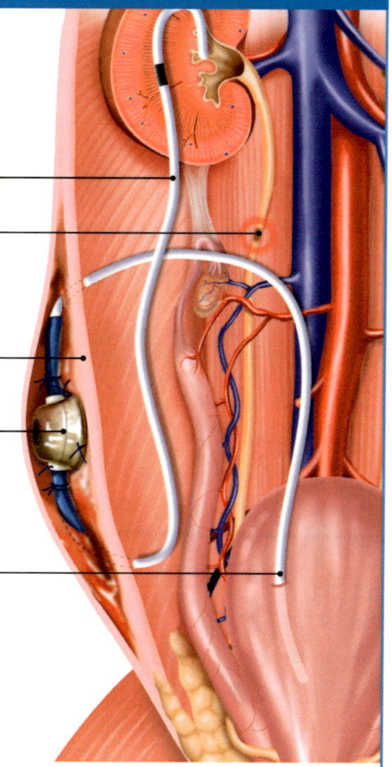

- This is a device that "bypasses" the ureter by creating a new tube from the affected kidney to the bladder.
- Part of its route runs outside the abdomen, in the subcutaneous plane.

Advantages:

- Allows urine samples to be taken from the renal pelvis for culture.

Complications:

- Short-term: leaks, semi-obstruction due to bent catheters or clots, bleeding during nephrostomy.
- Long-term: recurrent infections, dysuria, occlusion due to mineralisation, kinked catheters.

RENAL AND URINARY SYSTEM

18 Polycystic kidney disease (PKD)

This disease is hereditary and causes the formation of cysts in the kidneys. They are present from birth and, although they are initially very small, they grow over time and damage the kidney (kidney disease). They sometimes also affect the liver.

Breeds with a high risk: Persian, Exotic Shorthair, British Shorthair and crossbreeds of these breeds.

Breeds with a moderate risk: Birman, Burmilla, Devon Rex and Ragdoll.

Other breeds: very low risk.

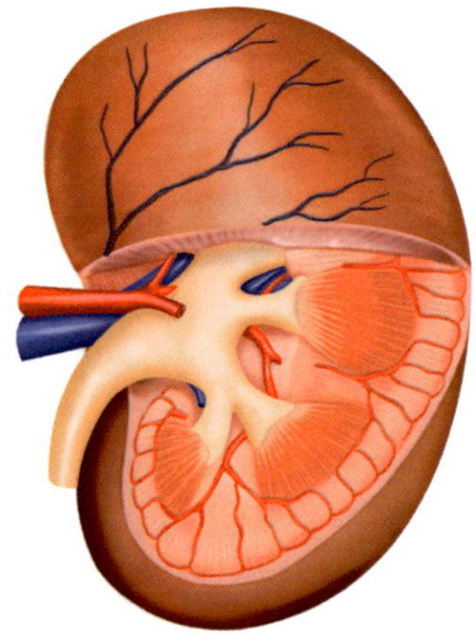

Normal kidney

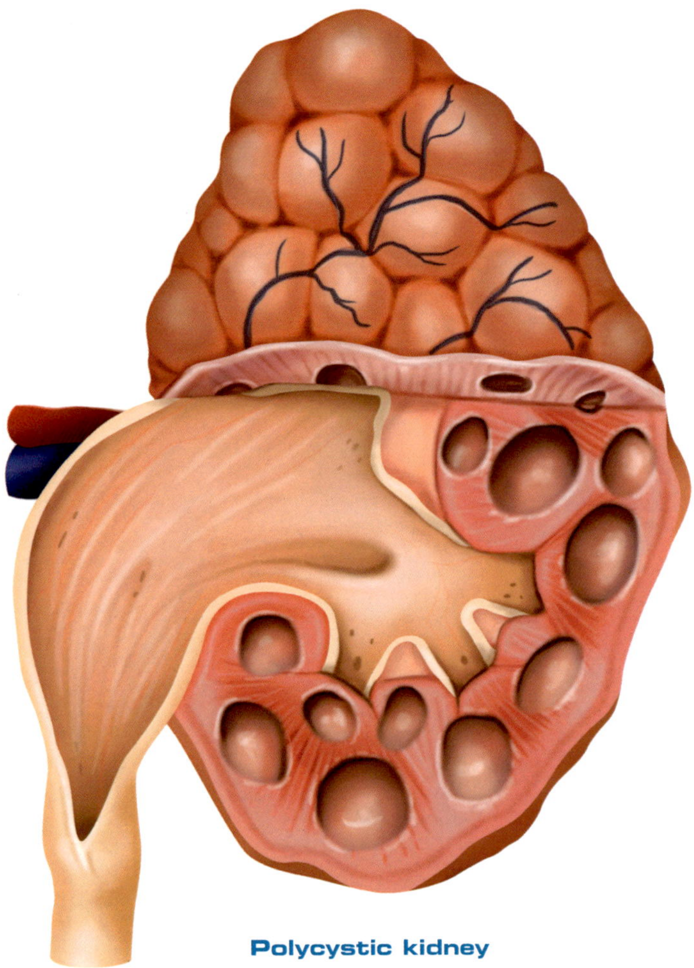

Polycystic kidney

Renal cysts

- Number: varies in each individual (from 20 to 200 cysts).
- Growth: it may be very fast (early death), or slow with symptoms of kidney disease from 8 years of age.
- Diagnosis:
  - Abdominal ultrasound.
  - Genetic testing with blood and saliva.

There are no treatments to prevent the progressive growth of cysts. Their growth speed is different in each cat and is determined by serial ultrasound studies.

Medical treatment

Necessary in cats who develop kidney disease.

Form of heredity

- It is transmitted by a single dominant autosomal gene; any cat with this gene will develop the disease.
- All the carriers of this gene are affected, even if they have few cysts.
- All the cats with the disease will transmit it to some of their offspring (approximately 50 %).

RENAL AND URINARY SYSTEM

19 Feline lower urinary tract disease (FLUTD)

Obstructive and non-obstructive

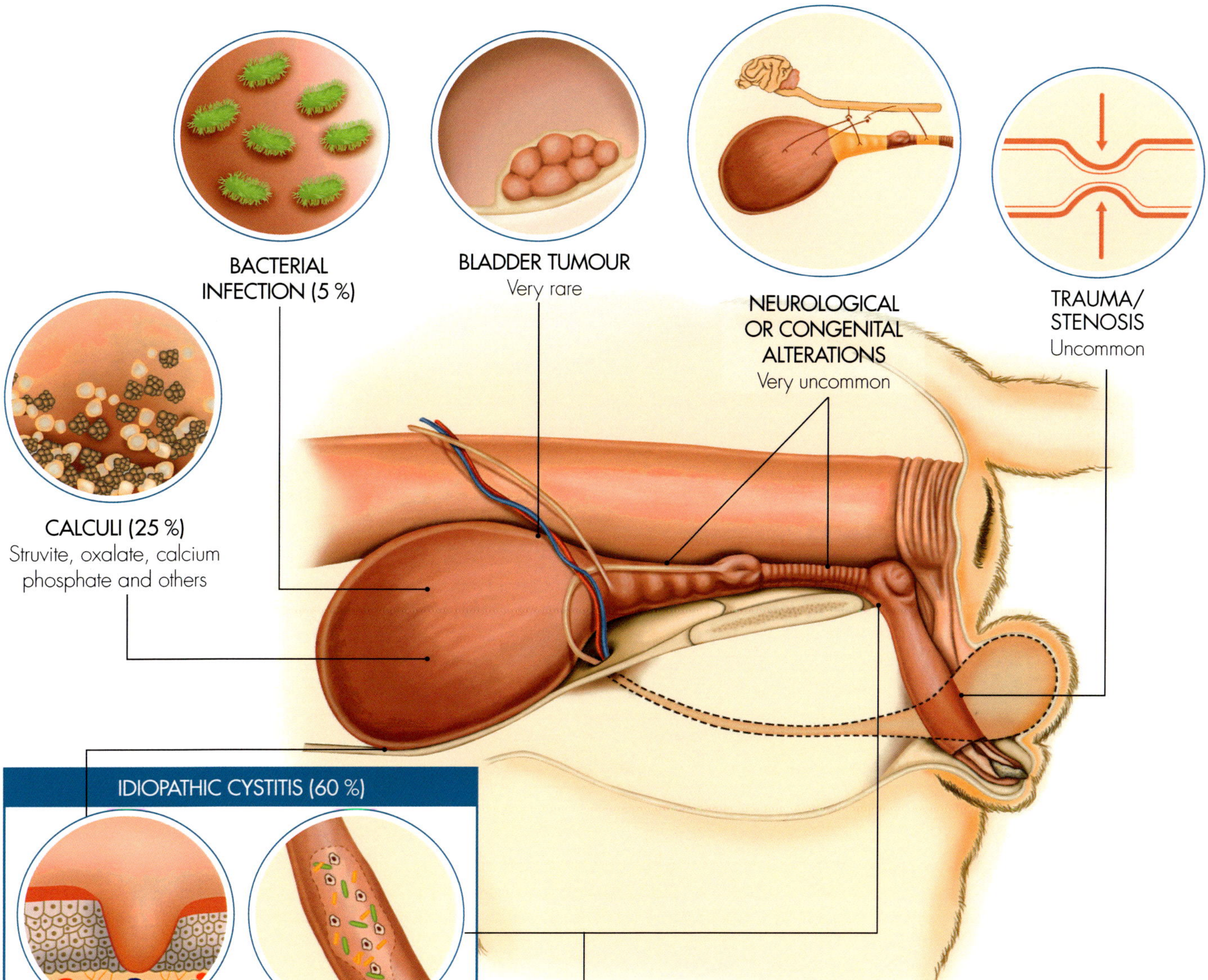

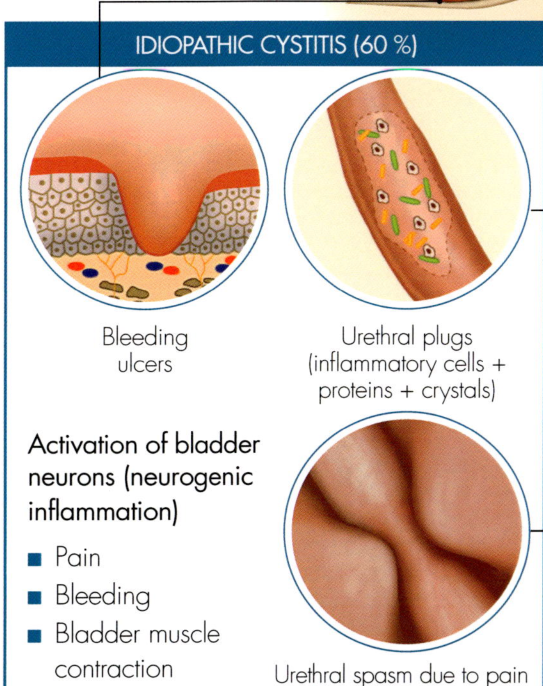

Clinical signs

- Difficulty in and pain during micturition.
- Affected animals frequently go to their litter tray to urinate.
- Blood may be observed in their urine.
- They may stop urinating in their tray due to pain.
- In case of obstructive FLUTD, inability to urinate due to urethral obstruction.

The cause of FLUTD must always be diagnosed to administer the appropriate treatment and prevent future recurrences.

RENAL AND URINARY SYSTEM

20 Perineal urethrostomy

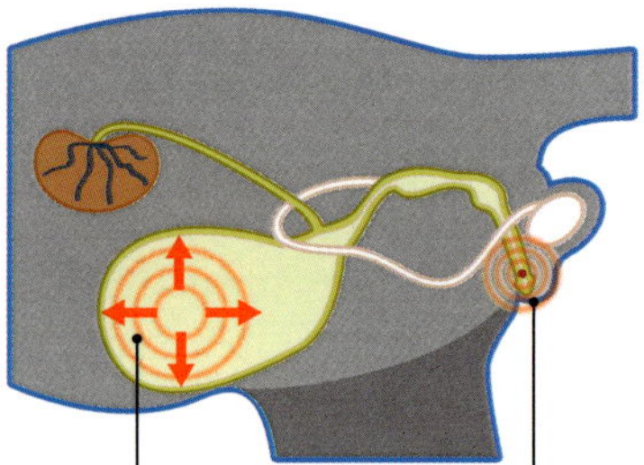

It involves creating an opening in the urethra and suturing it directly to the skin, in the perineal area below the anus, and removing the penis and testicles (if the cat is not already neutered).

Indications

- If the animal suffers from multiple obstructions (more than 3) despite treating FLUTD.
- Urethral obstruction impossible to resolve by means of catheterisation.
- Urethral stenosis.
- Severe penile injury.

Most complete urinary tract obstructions in cats are due to urethral plugs or to calculi.

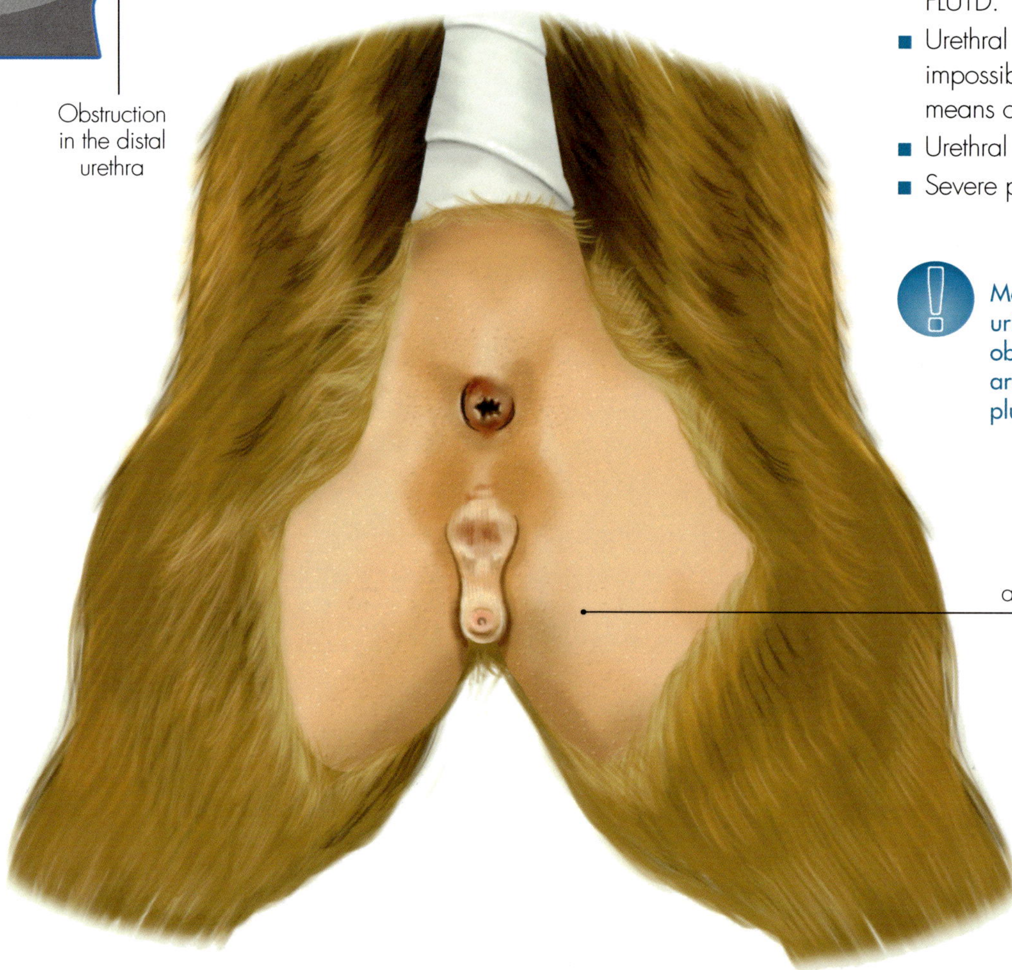

Surgical technique

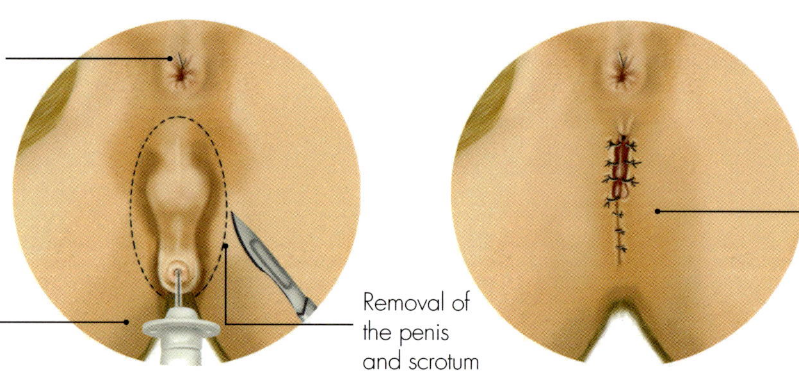

REPRODUCTIVE SYSTEM

21 The oestrus cycle in female cats

Female cats are seasonally polyoestrous females, whose cycles are stimulated by an increasing photoperiod. They have regular cycles during the months of the year with longer periods of light (from February–March to October–November). Some females may also cycle all year round if they are exposed to artificial light.

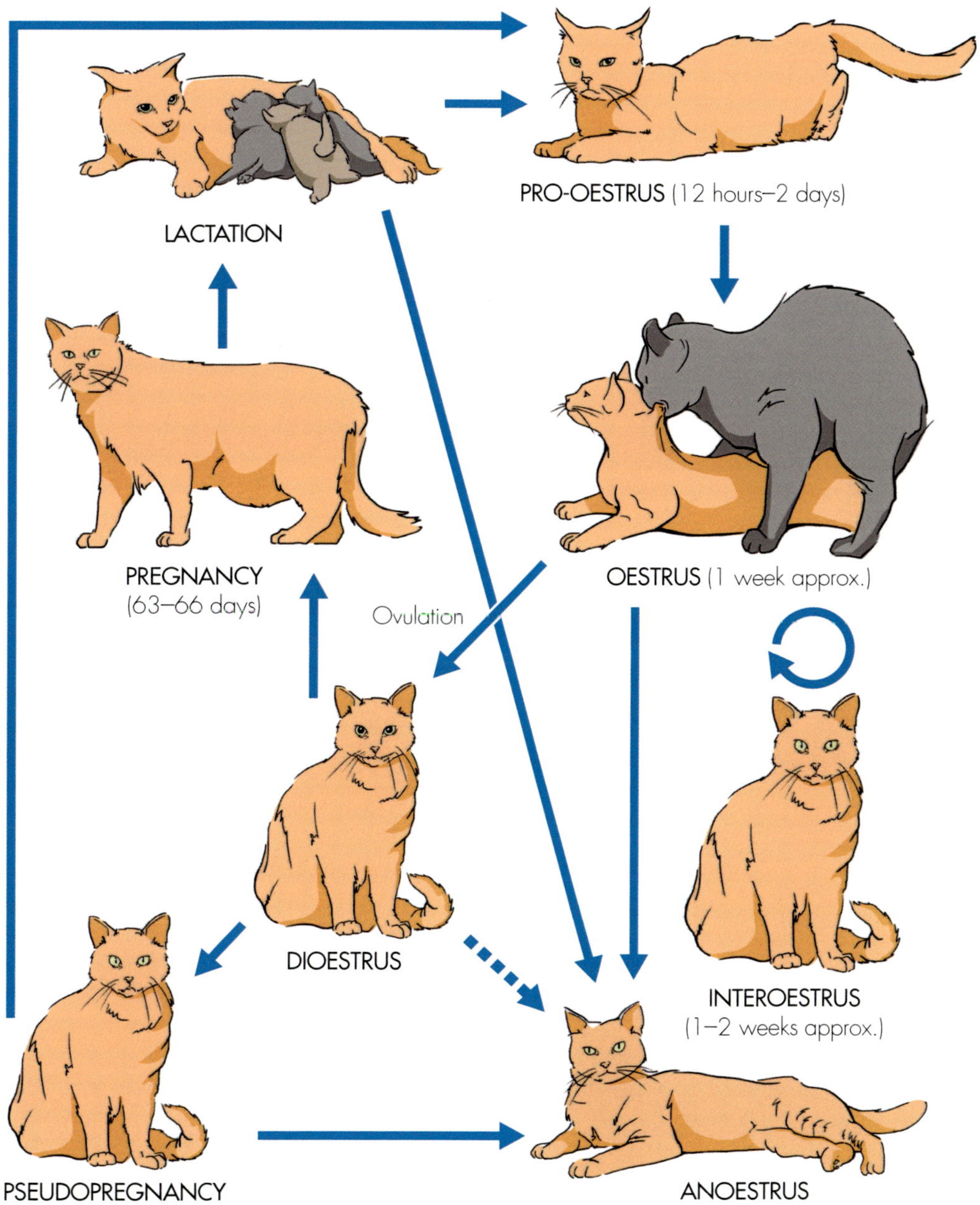

PRO-OESTRUS

- Males are attracted by non-receptive females.
- Mild vulvar oedema, with no bleeding (slight mucoid secretion).
- Sexual behaviour: purring, incessant meowing, lordosis behaviour, but does not allow mating.

OESTRUS

- Sexual behaviour similar to that of pro-oestrus, but the female allows mating.
- Ovulation induced by copulation. It may also be spontaneous.

INTEROESTRUS

- Appears when ovulation does not occur.
- Phase of inactivity between two consecutive heat cycles.

DIOESTRUS

- If ovulation takes place, the corpus luteum is formed (progesterone).
- Two situations may occur:
  - Pseudopregnancy: the cat ovulates, but there is no fertilisation.
  - Pregnancy: the cat ovulates and there is fertilisation.

ANOESTRUS

- Period with no sexual activity (absence of oestrus cycles).
- Between October–November and January–February (shorter periods of light). It may not appear under artificial light conditions.

They reach puberty between 6–8 months of age, although it may vary (4–12 months) depending on the weight, breed, etc.

The use of hormonal treatments to inhibit heat cycles should be avoided during the pro-oestrus and oestrus phases.
The moment of choice is usually the anoestrus phase.

REPRODUCTIVE SYSTEM

22 Neutering

in females and males

Female

Laparoscopic oophorectomy

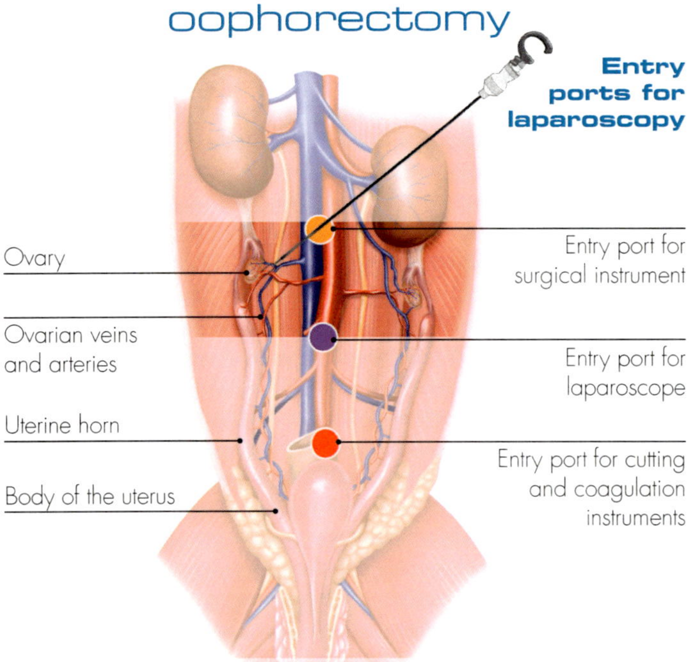

Laparoscopy is a minimally invasive technique that allows neutering through minimal incisions without exposing tissues.

Ovariohysterectomy via open surgery

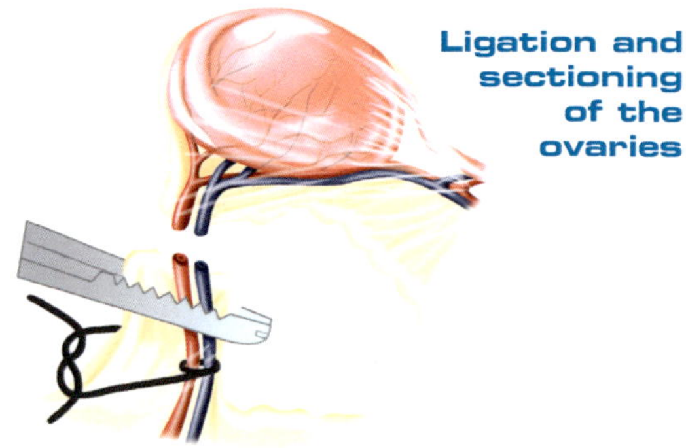

Double ligation and sectioning of the uterus

Removal of the uterus is recommended in females that have been in heat or had hydrometra, mucometra, etc.

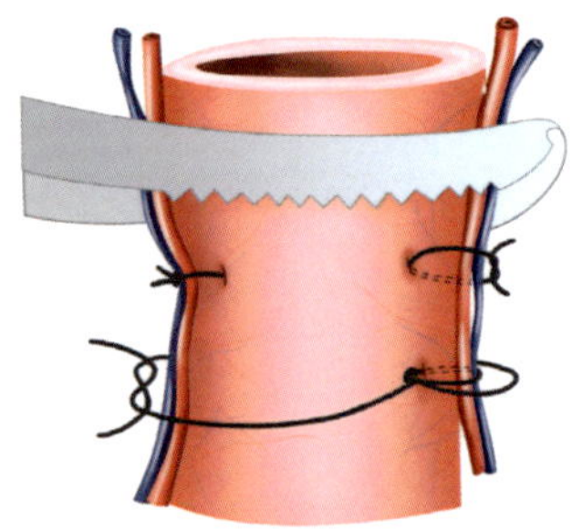

Male

Orchiectomy

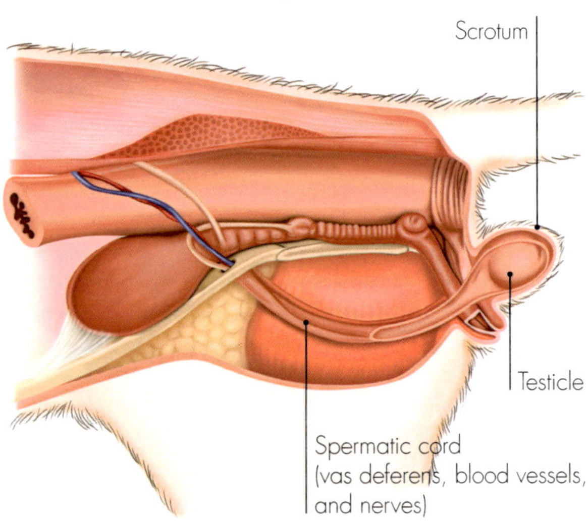

Once the testicle has been extracted from the scrotum, the spermatic cord is cut.

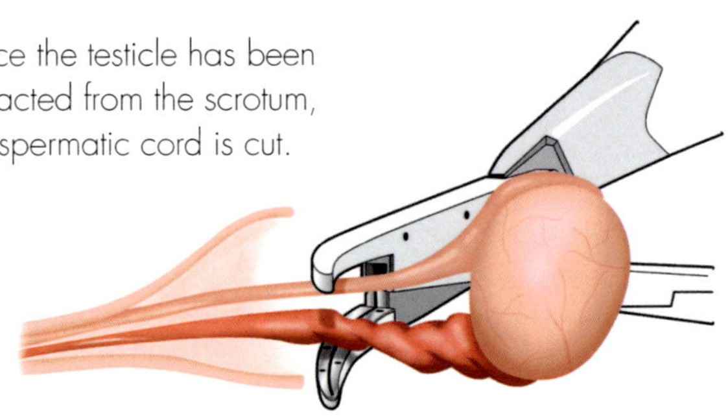

This can be achieved using a specialised instrument for separation and ligation, avoiding the need for sutures.

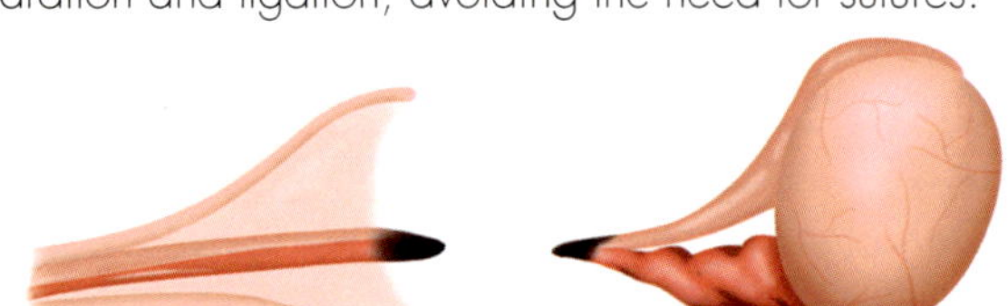

REPRODUCTIVE SYSTEM

23 Pyometra

Infection of the uterus

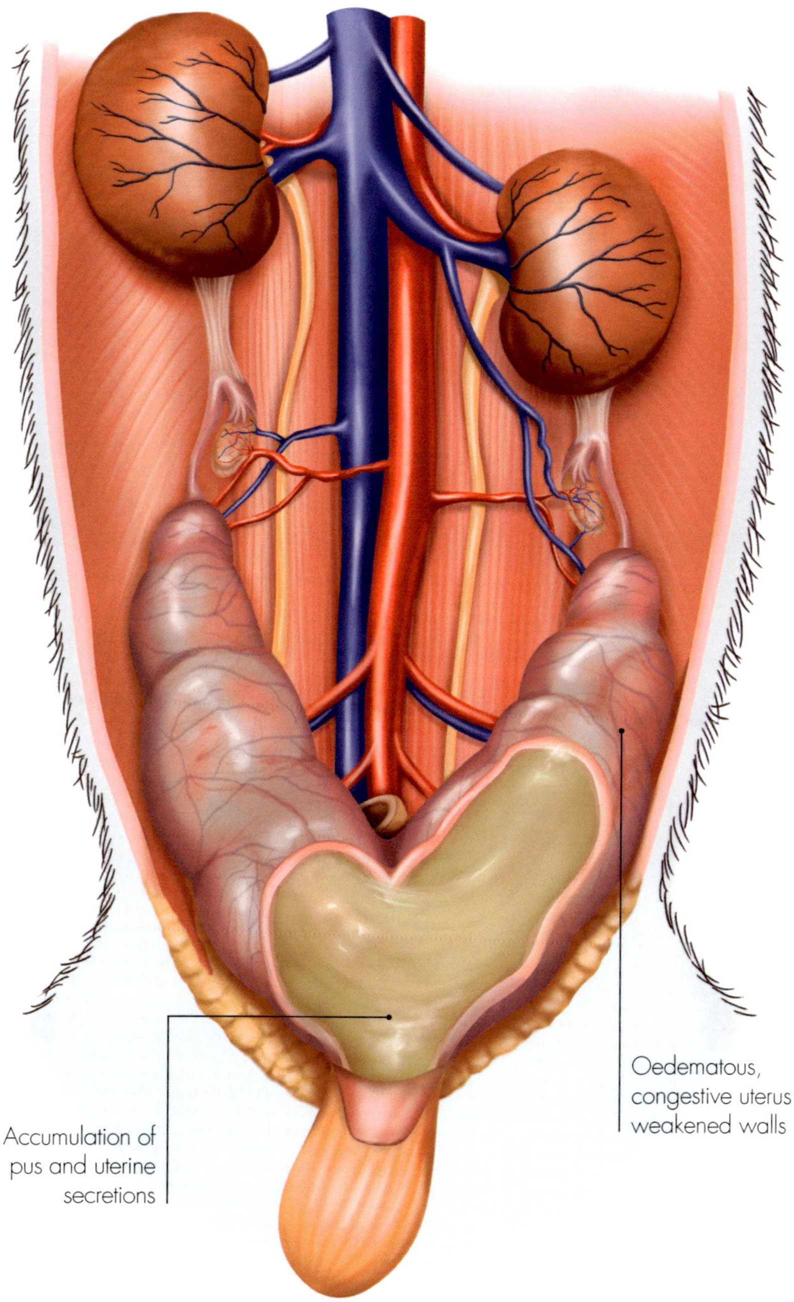

Infectious disease caused by bacteria and characterised by the presence of pus within the uterine cavity. It occurs in female cats of any age, regardless of whether they have already had kittens. The use of progestogens to inhibit oestrus is a risk factor.

Its diagnosis requires the use of abdominal radiography and ultrasonography.

Clinical signs

- Serous-bloody or mucopurulent vaginal discharge. If it is a closed-cervix pyometra, no secretions will be observed.
- Lethargy.
- Loss of weight.
- Polyuria and polydipsia.
- Fever is not common.

Medical treatment

- Fluid therapy.
- Antibiotics.
- Hormones until its resolution.

Surgical treatment

Treatment of choice (ovariohysterectomy), especially if it is not a breeding female and if signs of severe infection such as peritonitis are observed.

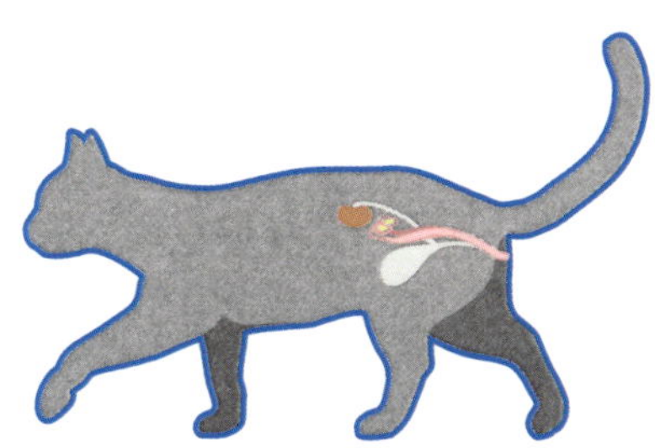

REPRODUCTIVE SYSTEM

24 Residual ovary syndrome

This syndrome should be suspected when cats continue to show signs of heat after sterilisation. Surgical treatment is required to locate and remove the remaining ovarian tissue.

Causes

- Presence of ectopic ovarian tissue.
- Autotransplantation of ovarian tissue.
- Failure of the surgical procedure.

Diagnosis

- Presence of the usual signs of heat.
- Vaginal cytology during clinical signs compatible with oestrus.
- Chorionic gonadotropin stimulation test.
- Diagnostic imaging: ultrasound will enable detection of ovarian tissue, which will be hypoechoic and contain cystic structures. However, failure to detect tissue does not rule out its presence.
- Exploratory or laparoscopic laparotomy.

Exploratory laparotomy and laparoscopy allow diagnosis and treatment by removing ovarian tissue.

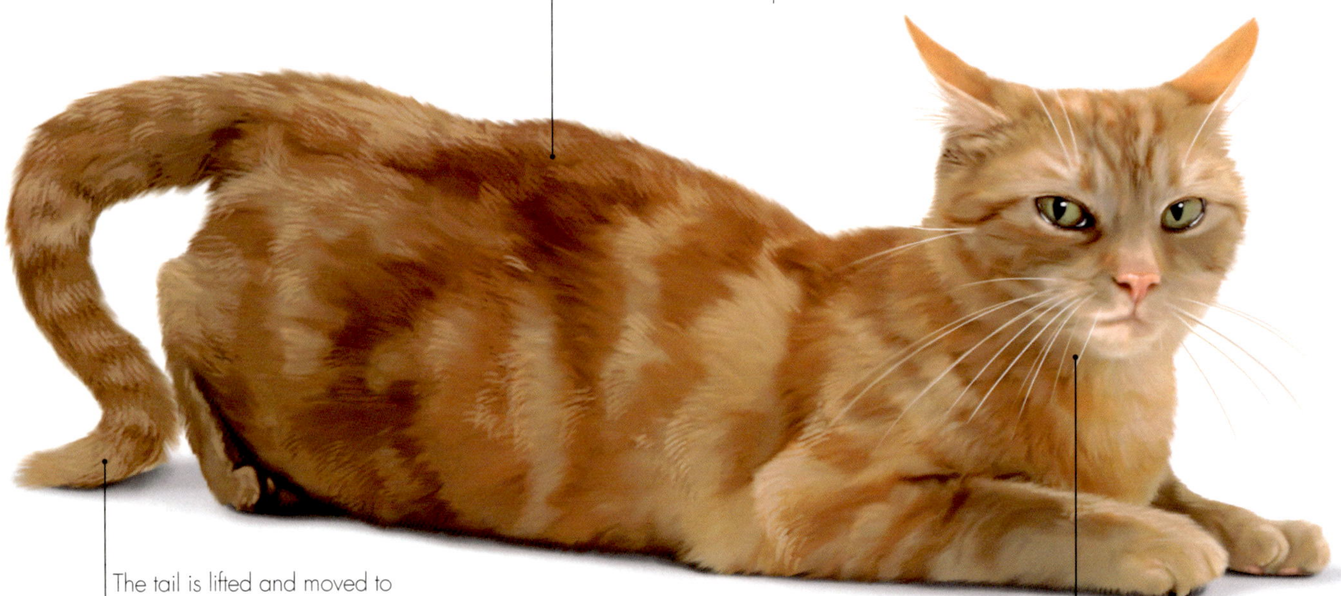
Posture typical of cat in heat, with the anterior third lowered and the posterior third raised
The tail is lifted and moved to display the area of the vulva
Purring and meowing increase

REPRODUCTIVE SYSTEM

25 Mammary tumours

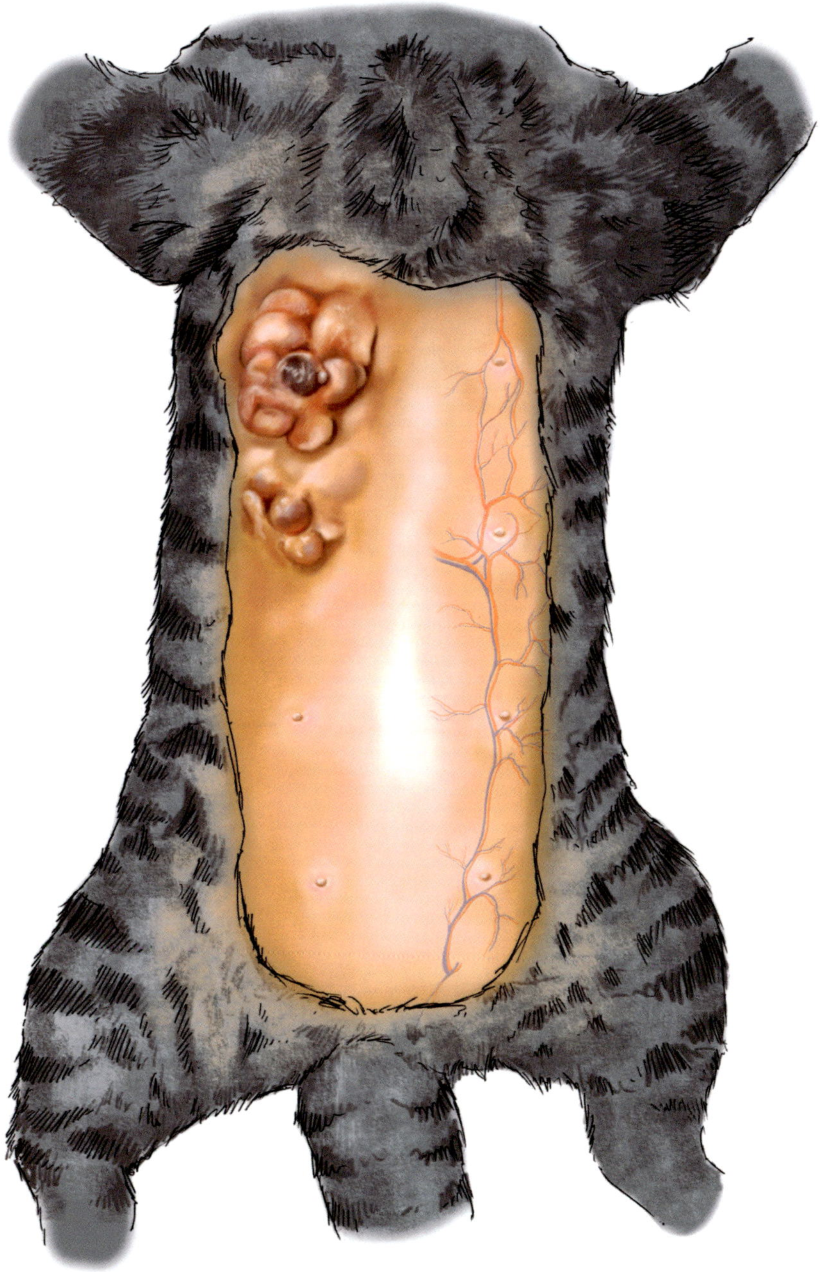

In cats, 80–96 % of mammary tumours are malignant, the most frequent ones being tubular and papillary adenocarcinomas. Barely 10 % of cases are adenomas. Only 1–2 % of mammary tumours occur in males. The average age of presentation is 11 years, although it may affect younger female cats. The diagnosis of mammary tumours requires a biopsy, and thoracic radiography and abdominal ultrasonography to rule out the presence of metastases.

The risk of carcinoma is 6–7 times lower in females neutered before 6 months of age.

Clinical signs

Size is the most important factor:

- One or several firm, lobulated masses, which are occasionally ulcerated if they are large.
- Frequent local glandular involvement.
- Metastases in the lung and organs such as the liver and lymph nodes, very common in nodules >3 cm.

The use of progestogens to control oestrus cycles increases the risk of developing mammary tumours or adenomatous hyperplasia.

Prognosis

Size is the most important factor:

- Female cats with tumours <2 cm may live up to 3 years after the surgery.
- Cats with tumours <3 cm live for about 4–6 months.

Surgical treatment

Radical surgery, removing the entire mammary chain, reduces the risk of recurrence (relapse).

Medical treatment

Chemotherapy may increase the interval between relapses as well as life expectancy.

CARDIORESPIRATORY SYSTEM

26 Brachycephaly in cats

The brachycephalic conformation of the skull in Persian and Himalayan cats causes obstruction of the upper airways, disorders of the tear drainage system and alters the structure of the teeth. The more brachycephalic their skull is, the more severe these signs will be.

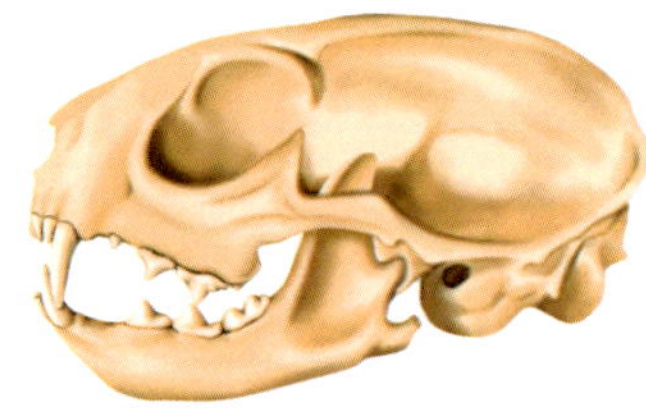

Normal skull

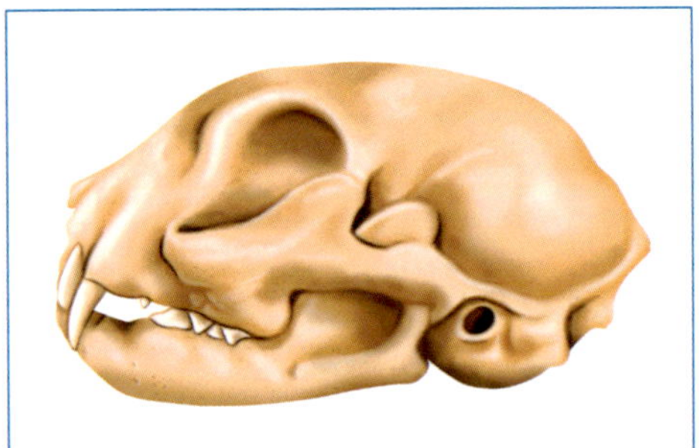

Grade I: mild

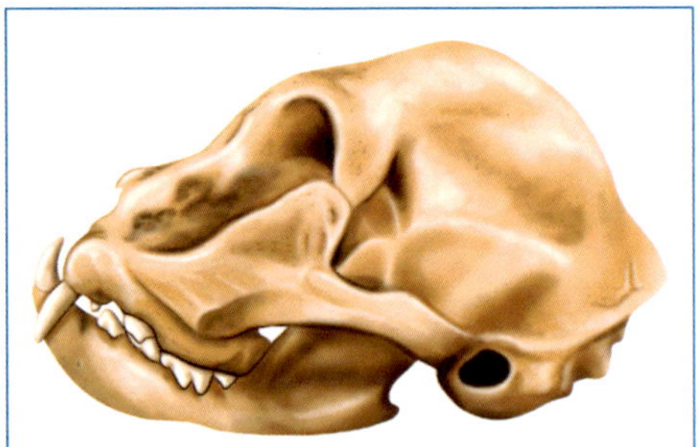

Grade II: moderate

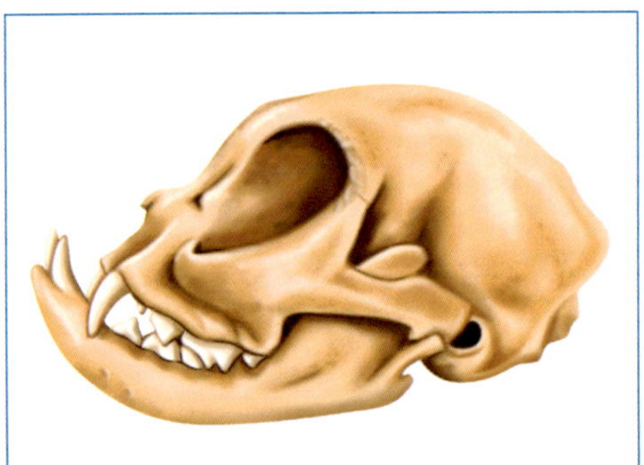

Grade III: intense

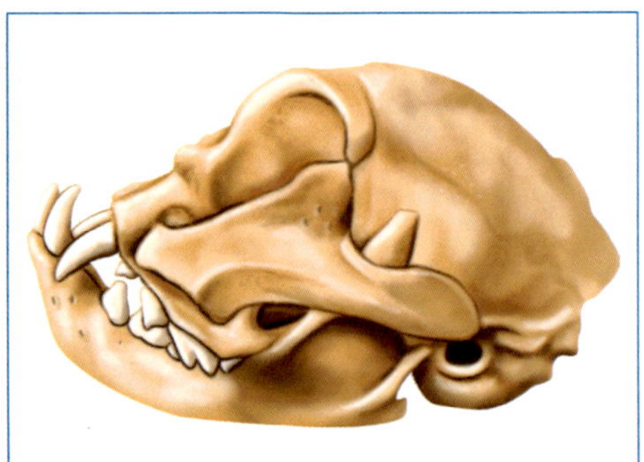

Grade IV: severe

Clinical signs

The higher the degree of brachycephaly, the more severe the signs will be:

- Alteration of the tear duct: constant tearing and secondary dermatitis.
- Greater exposure of the eyes: keratitis and corneal sequestra.
- Incorrect teeth alignment: difficulties in chewing and more frequent periodontal disease.
- Obstruction of the upper airways due to:
  - Stenotic nares.
  - Narrow nasal cavity.
  - Elongated soft palate.

Medical treatment

- In case of dermatitis of skinfolds due to epiphora.
- In case of keratitis.

Surgical treatment

- Surgical correction of stenotic nares and elongated soft palate.
- Removal of the teeth that prevent proper chewing.

Recommendations

The international veterinary community recommends the prohibition to breed cats with extreme brachycephaly due to the negative consequences on their health and life expectancy.

CARDIORESPIRATORY SYSTEM

27 Nasopharyngeal polyps

These are benign masses that can occur at any age, although their frequency is higher in young cats. They originate in the epithelium of the tympanic bulla or in the Eustachian tube: they are known as aural polyps if they grow into the ear canal and nasopharyngeal polyps if they grow into the nasopharynx. In this case, the tympanic bullae are affected by inflammatory tissue produced by obstruction of the Eustachian tube, and not by growth of the polyp. Growth towards the nasopharynx and towards the ear is uncommon.

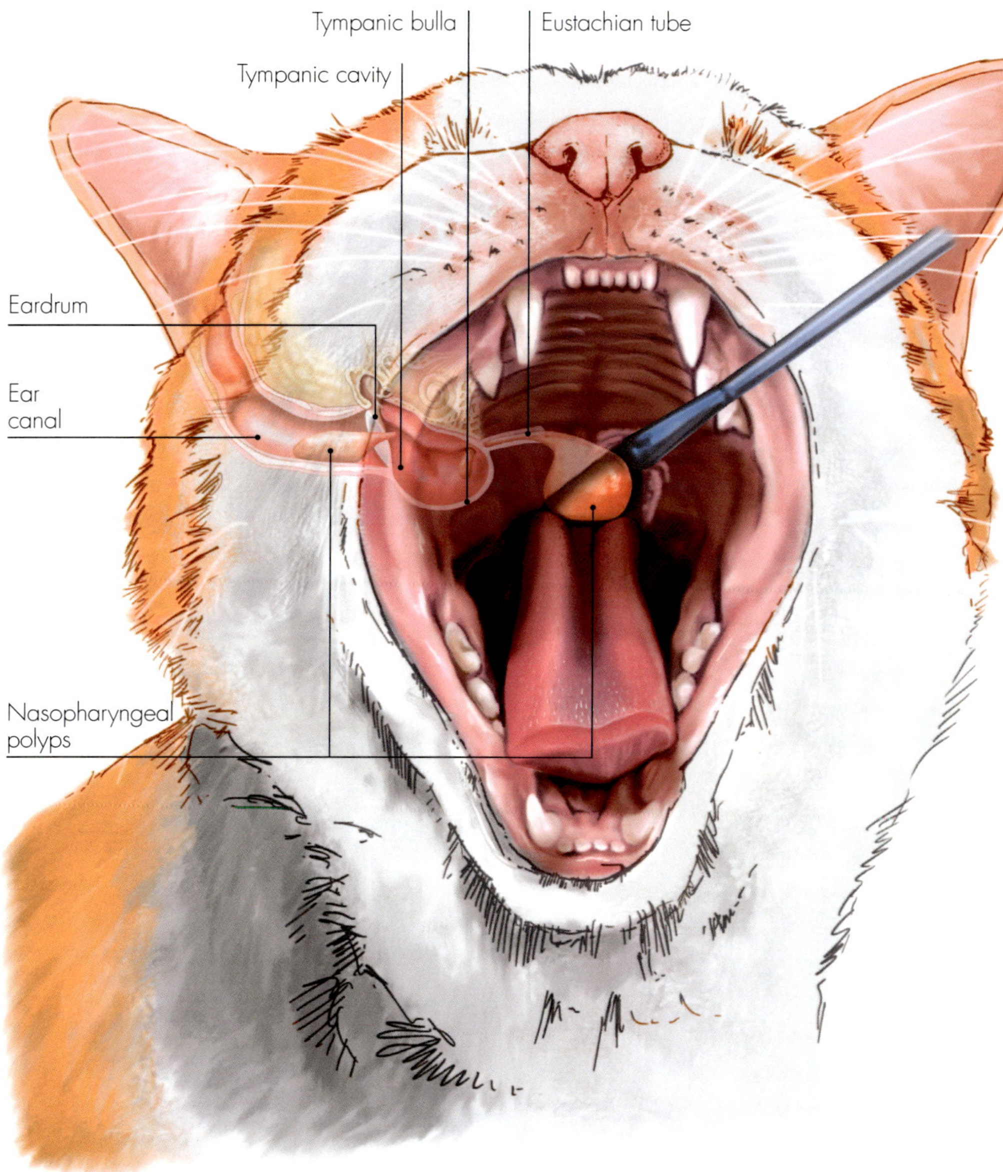

They are secondary to inflammatory or infectious processes of the respiratory tract or middle ear.

Clinical signs

- They are chronic and progressive, and affect the airways or inner ear.
- Respiratory:
  - Rhinitis and sinusitis with chronic nasal secretion and sneezing.
  - Dysphagia, cyanosis and syncope in case of obstruction of the airways.
- In the inner ear:
  - Otitis externa, media or interna, depending on their extension, with ear secretion, head tilt, nystagmus, vestibular ataxia and Horner's syndrome.

Diagnosis

- Radiography of the nasopharynx.
- Evaluation of tympanic bullae by computed tomography (CT).

Treatment

- Nasopharyngeal polyps: surgery by traction/avulsion of the polyp from the nasopharynx provides good results.
- Aural polyps: require ventral osteotomy of the bulla.

CARDIORESPIRATORY SYSTEM

28 Hypertrophic cardiomyopathy

Cardiomyopathy is more frequent in cats. It may be primary or secondary to hyperthyroidism, hypertension, obstruction of the outflow tract, acromegaly or myocardial neoplasia, and these conditions must therefore be ruled out. There may not be any clinical signs until it is very advanced, which is why an early diagnosis by means of echocardiography is essential.

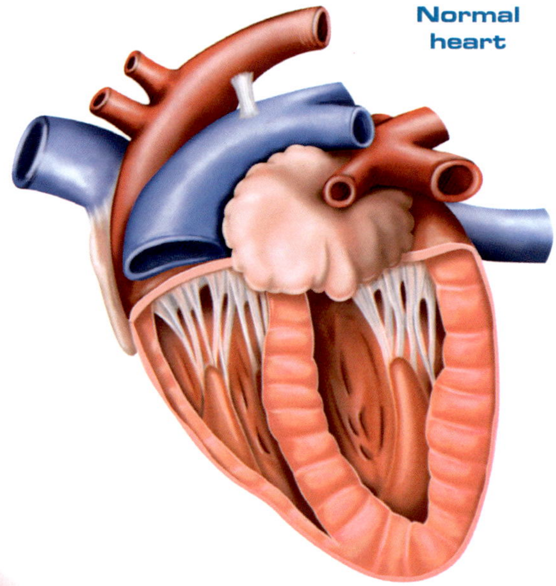

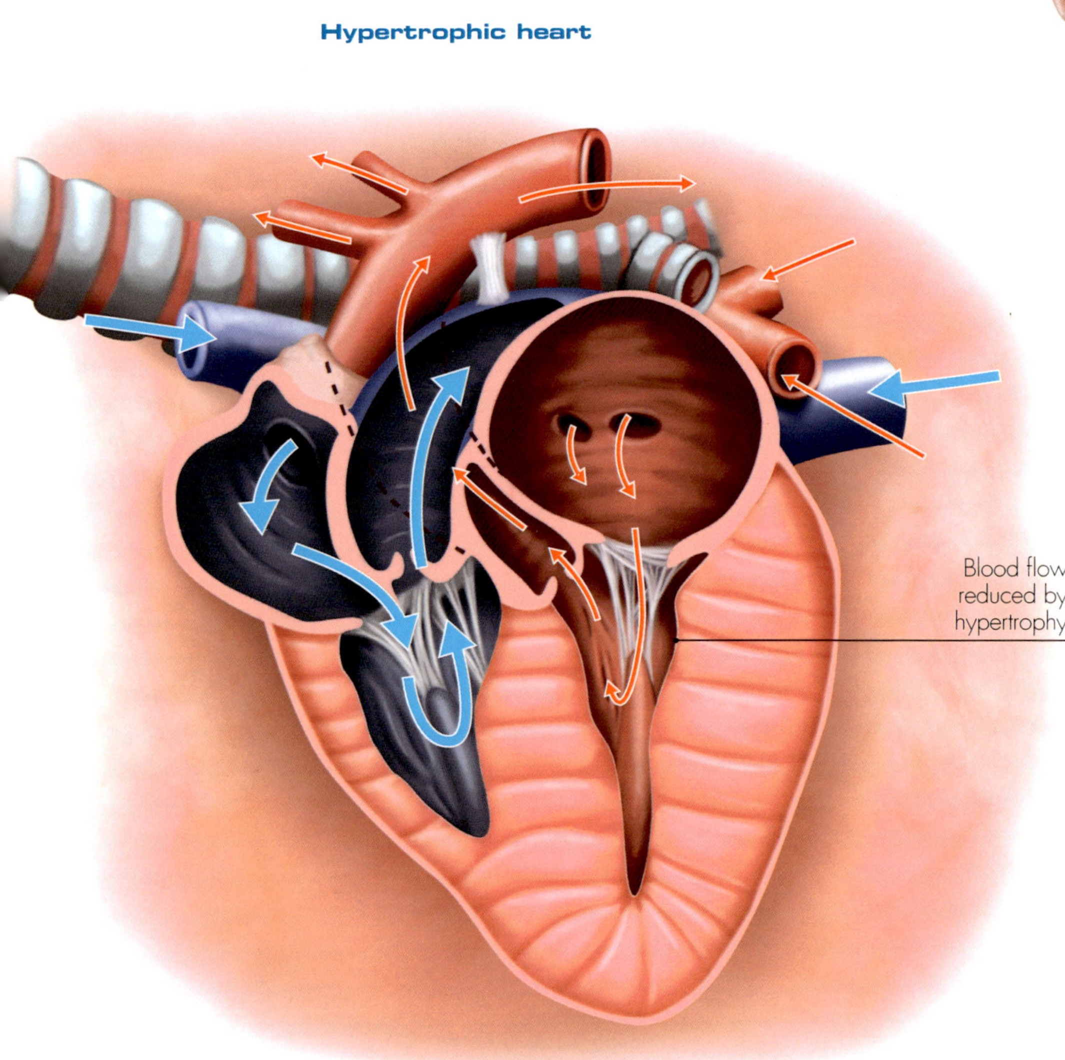

It affects almost all the breeds, although there is a genetic predisposition in the Maine Coon, Ragdoll, Norwegian Forest and British Shorthair.

The left ventricle cannot be filled properly due to the hypertrophy of its wall (diastolic dysfunction).

Medical treatment

Each stage requires a different type of treatment and no specific treatment is currently recommended at very early stages.

Clinical signs

- Murmur (approx. 60 % of cats with cardiomyopathy).
- Galloping rhythm.
- Limb paralysis caused by aortic thromboembolism (7 % of cats).
- Acute respiratory distress due to pulmonary oedema and/or pleural effusion.

CARDIORESPIRATORY SYSTEM

29 Restrictive cardiomyopathy

Restrictive cardiomyopathy is the most common myocardial condition after hypertrophic cardiomyopathy. It can be primary, caused by myocarditis and viral inflammation, or secondary, as occurs in the final stages of hypertrophic cardiomyopathy, valvular disease, or myocardial infarction. It is usually diagnosed when patients present with signs of congestive heart failure.

Ultrasound signs

- Dilation of the left atrium or of both atria may be observed.
- The myocardial thickness is normal or slightly increased.
- Fibrous bands are common.
- Fibrous tissue is observed in the interventricular septum, papillary muscles, or ventricular wall and may also be detected in the myocardium and endocardium.
- Pericardial effusion may occur in advanced cases.

Course

- The prognosis is poor as it progresses to congestive heart failure or thromboembolism.
- Survival time is usually less than 1 year.
- Sudden death can occur.

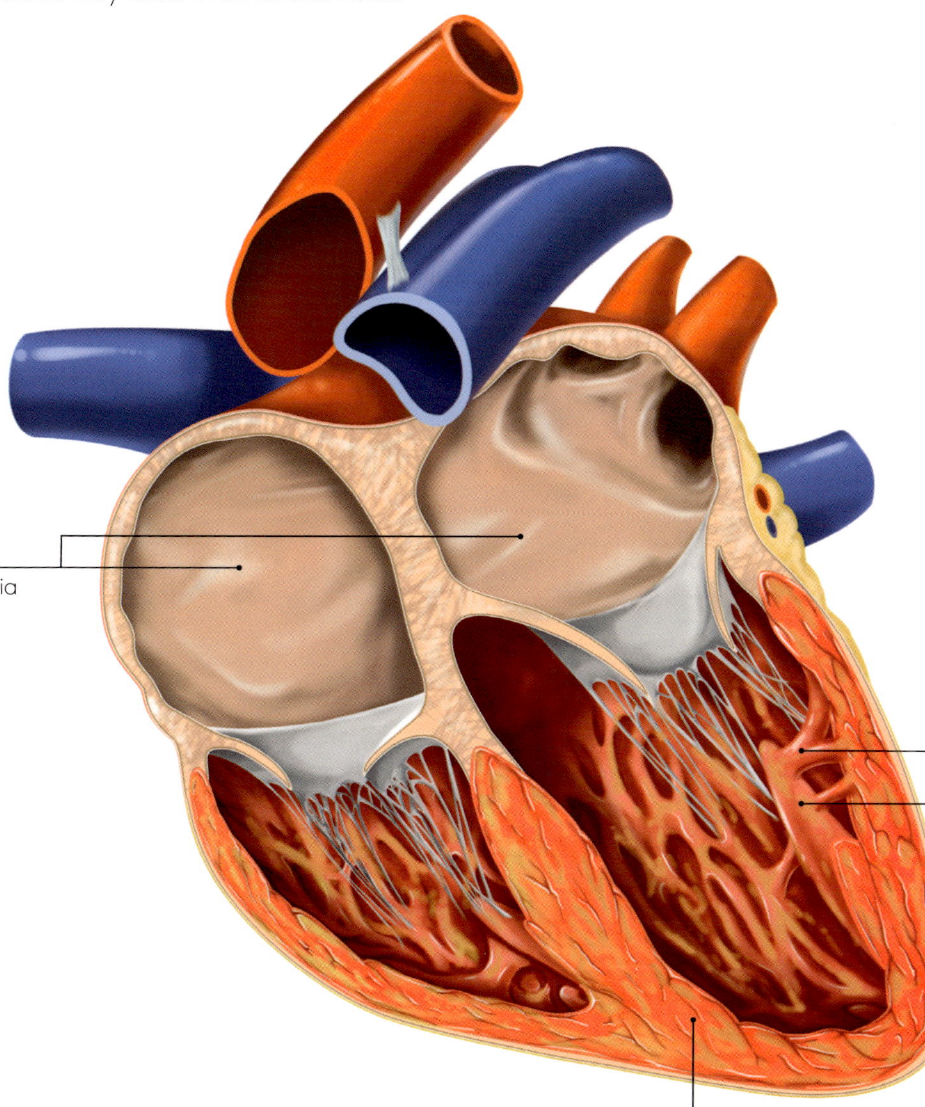

CARDIORESPIRATORY SYSTEM

30 Dilated cardiomyopathy

The anomalous dilation of the cardiac muscle may be originated by a deficiency in taurine (cats fed with dog food), be idiopathic (in most cases), or appear as the end stage of a non-diagnosed valvular disease or of a myocardial ischaemic disease.

Breed predisposition: Siamese, Burmese and Abyssinian.

Normal heart

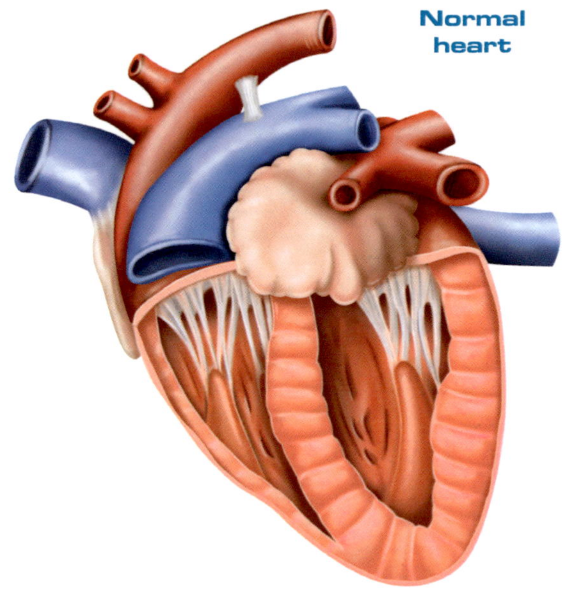

Dilated heart

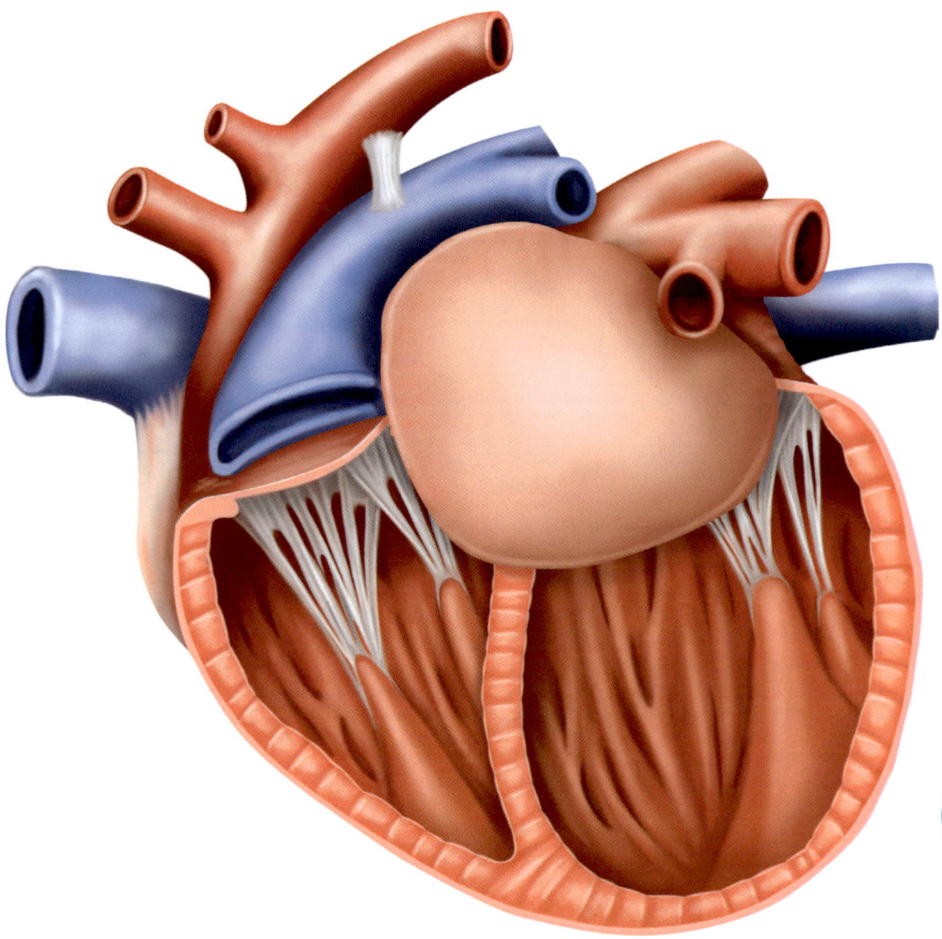

Clinical signs

- Murmur (approx. 60 % of cats with cardiomyopathy).
- Galloping rhythm.
- Limb paralysis caused by aortic thromboembolism (7 % of cats).
- Acute respiratory distress due to pulmonary oedema and/or pleural effusion.
- Progressive weight loss and weakness.

The animal may not show any signs until the disease is very advanced, which is why an early diagnosis by means of echocardiography is essential.

Medical treatment

Taurine levels should always be measured since its administration may correct the disease.

Taurine

- Essential amino acid for the normal functioning of the cardiac muscle, sight and reproduction, among other functions.
- Cats cannot synthesise it in a sufficient amount and must therefore obtain it from their diet.
- Its deficiency may cause: blindness, dilated cardiomyopathy, insufficient growth and poor reproductive results.

CARDIORESPIRATORY SYSTEM

31 Arterial thromboembolism

Frequent complication associated with all types of cardiomyopathy in cats. Other causes of thromboembolism are: arterial thrombosis due to a vascular lesion, infection or tumours (pulmonary carcinomas).

On rare occasions, the forelimbs, cerebral, renal or mesenteric arteries may be affected.

Clinical signs

- Acute excruciating pain.
- Paralysis or paresis of the affected limbs.
- The affected limbs do not have a pulse, are pale and cold.
- Some cats will also have signs of congestive heart failure.

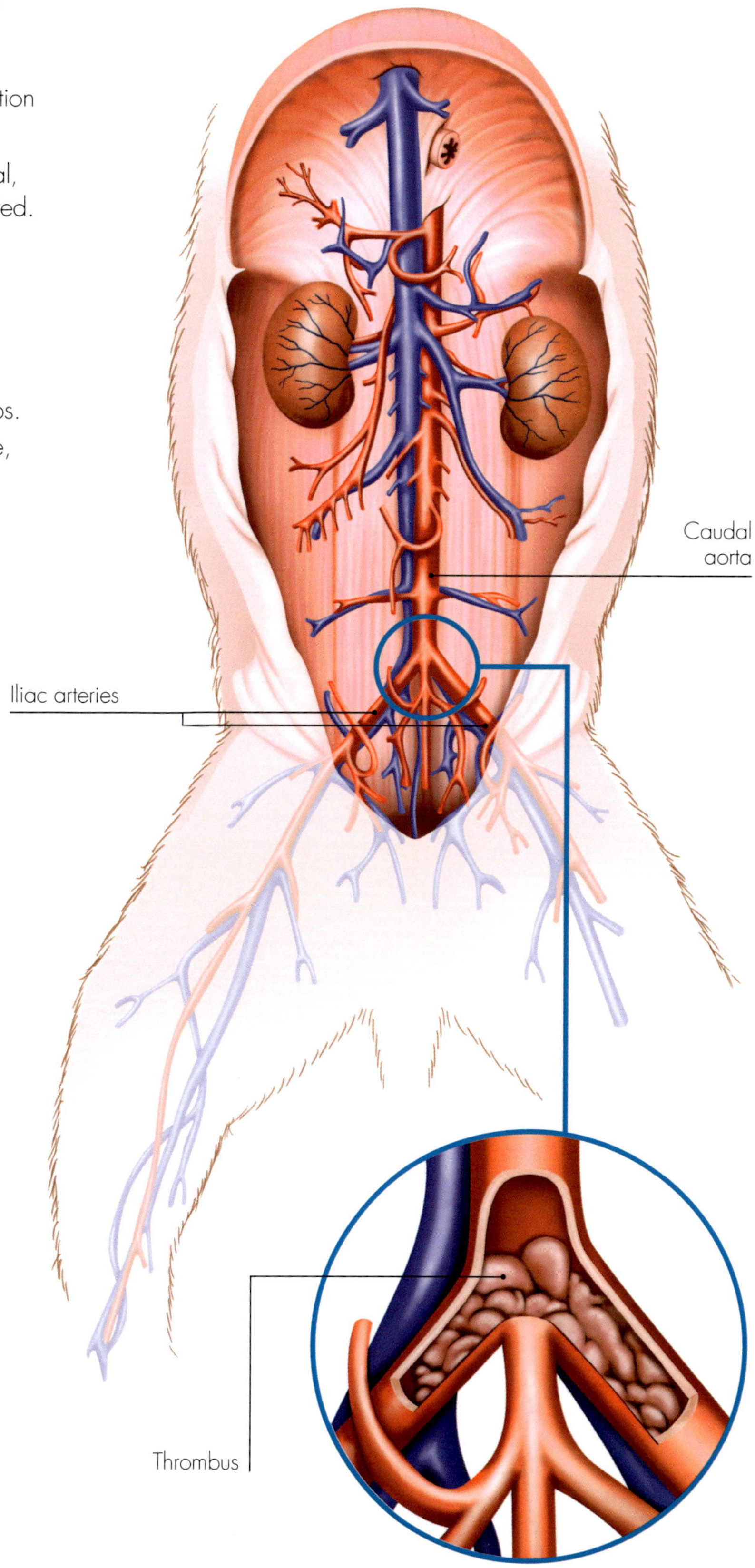

Prognosis

- Poor, since mortality is high.
- Cats with only one affected limb usually have a better prognosis.

Most thrombi are located at the bifurcation of the aorta, which causes paralysis of one or two hind limbs.

CARDIORESPIRATORY SYSTEM

32 Cough in cats

Multiple diseases cause cough in cats. The most common cause of cough is feline bronchial inflammatory disease, which groups two entities: bronchial asthma and chronic bronchitis.

Differential diagnosis

- Bacterial: *Mycoplasma* spp., *Bordetella bronchiseptica*.
- Parasitic: *Aelurostrongylus abstrusus, Toxoplasma gondii, Toxocara cati*.
- Viral: acute herpesvirus and calicivirus pneumonitis.
- Neoplastic: bronchial or bronchoalveolar carcinoma.
- Inflammatory bronchial disease:
  - Asthma.
  - Chronic bronchitis.

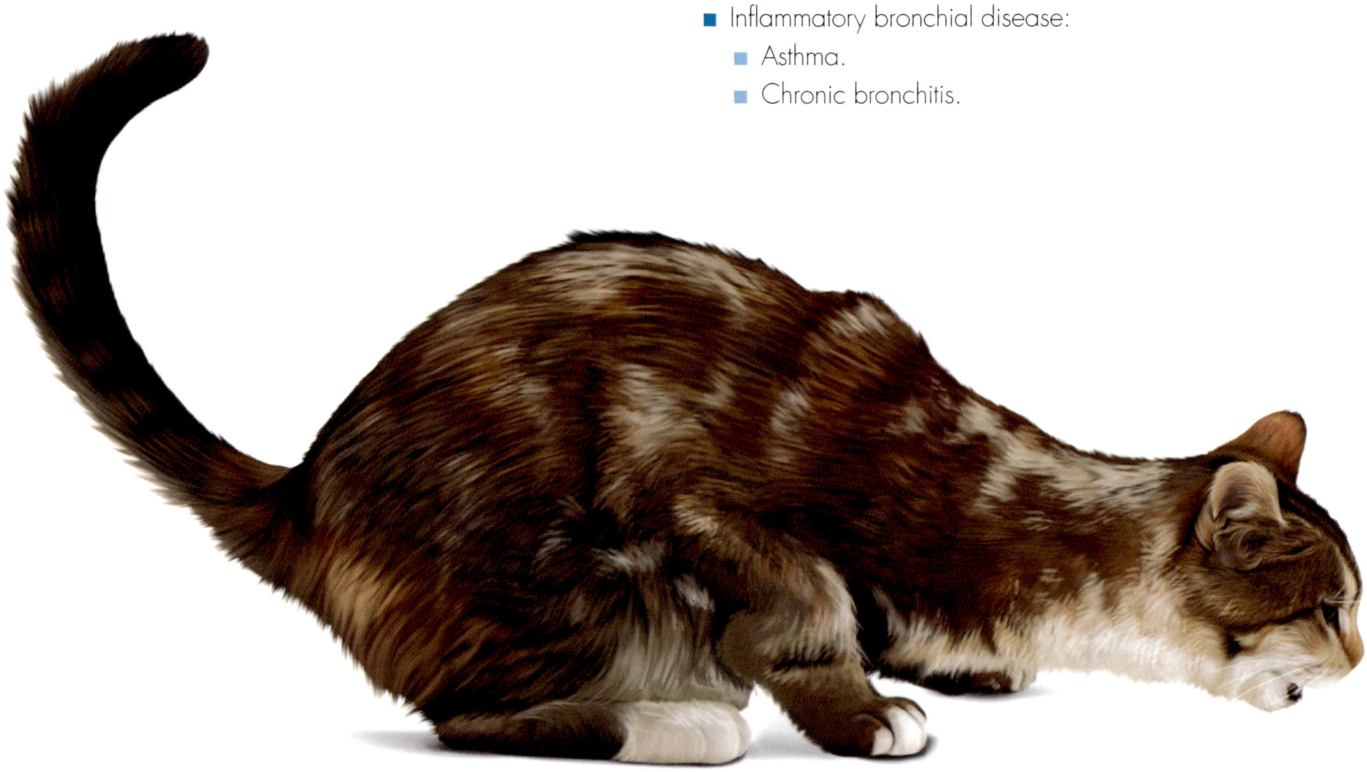

Diagnosis

Requires an orderly diagnostic approach:

- Chest radiography.
- Lung ultrasound.
- Rule out lung parasites.
- Bronchoalveolar lavage: performed by blind method or by bronchoscopy. Various tests are carried out on the samples obtained: cytology, culture, and PCR for *Mycoplasma* spp. This test allows differentiation between chronic bronchitis and asthmatic bronchitis.

Bronchoalveolar lavage is the essential test for the definitive diagnosis of chronic bronchitis or asthmatic bronchitis.

CARDIORESPIRATORY SYSTEM

33 Feline asthma

Feline asthma is the most common bronchial disease in cats. It occurs due to hypersensitivity reactions to inhaled allergens (dust, pollen, mites) or other factors (changes of temperature, drugs, exercise, infections, etc.), which cause chronic inflammation of the lower airways with an increase in the production of mucus and bronchoconstriction.

Diagnosis requires imaging techniques and bronchoalveolar lavage.

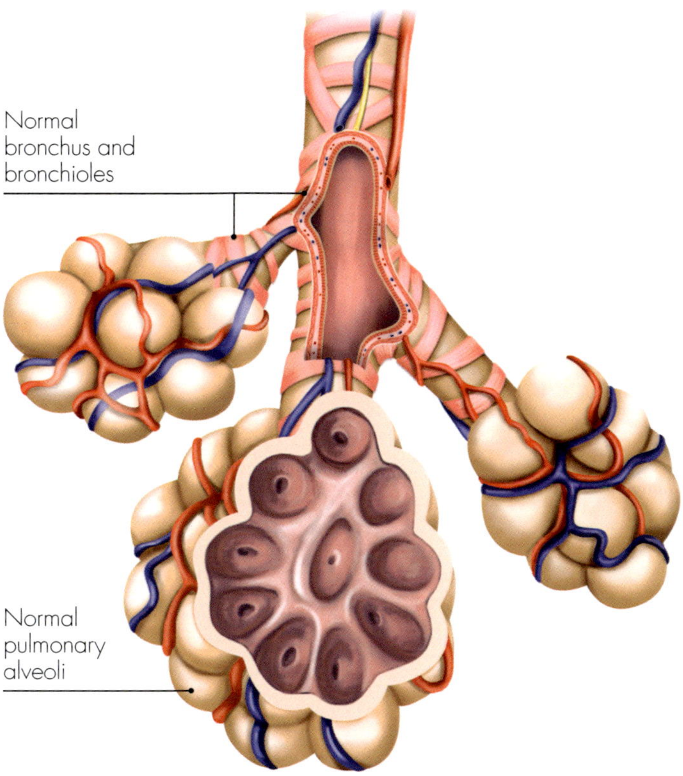

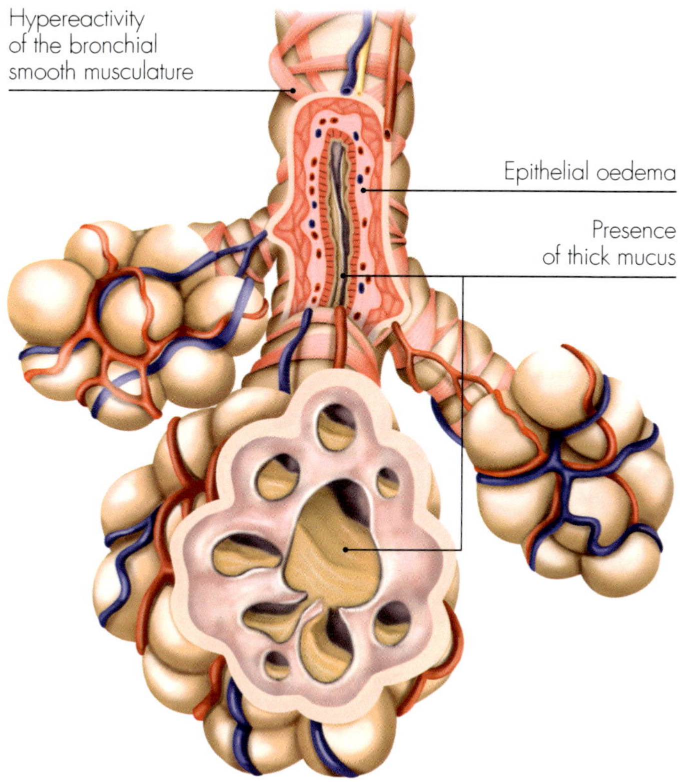

Clinical signs

- Chronic or intermittent cough with a variable intensity.
- Difficulty breathing due to acute bronchoconstriction in severe cases.

Medical treatment

- Corticosteroid inhalers, applied with a specific aerosol chamber for cats, are the treatment of choice.
- Immune therapy by means of a monthly vaccine against the responsible allergens may be successful in a great percentage of cases of asthma.

Recommendations

In order to avoid environmental irritating agents:

- Use clumping litter and discard closed trays with doors.
- Do not smoke or use sprays, incense or aerosol air fresheners.
- Vacuum clean regularly.

CARDIORESPIRATORY SYSTEM

34 Pneumothorax

Accumulation of air in the pleural space, which leads to severe and acute breathing difficulty (dyspnoea).

Types

- **Open:** defect in the thoracic wall, which allows outside air to enter the pleural space.
- **Closed:** air leaks from the lung, bronchi, caudal trachea or oesophagus into the pleural space.
- **Tension:** tear in the pleura, which lets air in at inspiration, but does not let it out at expiration.

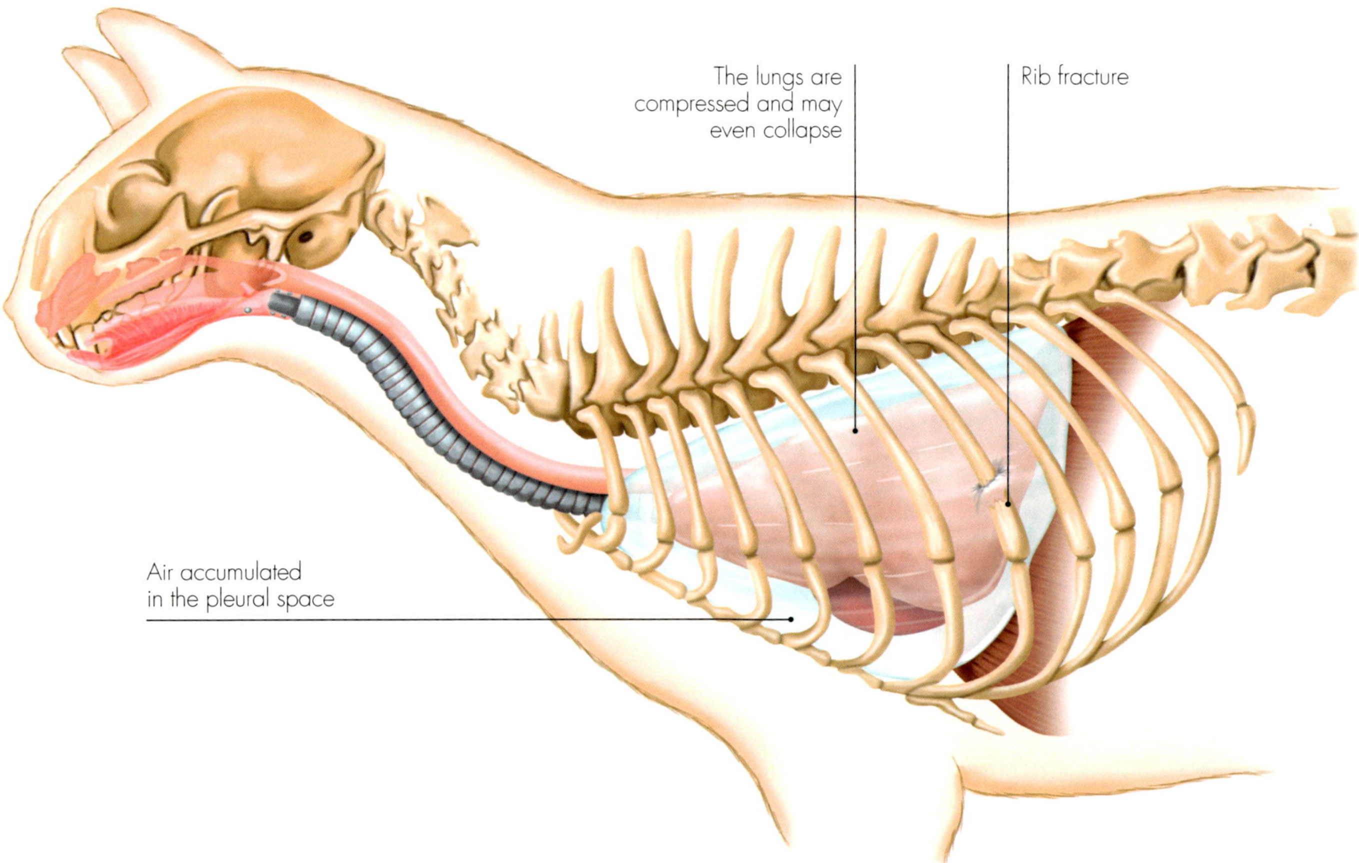

Medical treatment

- Oxygen chamber and analgesic treatment.
- Thoracocentesis and removal of air located in the pleural space.

Surgical treatment

Necessary on very few occasions.

It may be traumatic or spontaneous due to severe pulmonary disease (tumours, bronchopneumonia) leading to necrosis of the visceral pleura.

CARDIORESPIRATORY SYSTEM

35 Pleural effusion

It is the presence of fluid in the pleural space, which leads to progressive breathing difficulty.

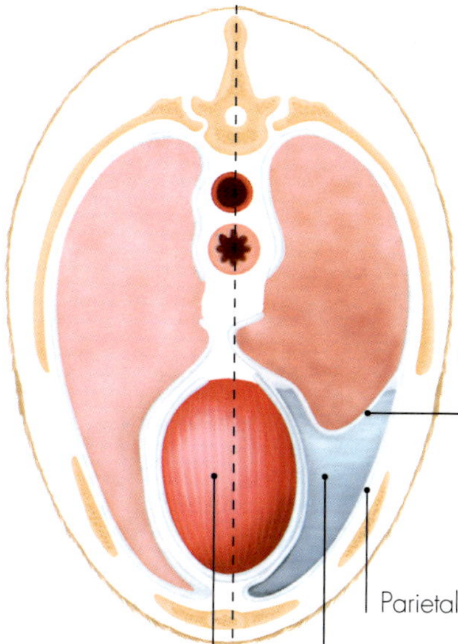

Types of fluid and causes

- **Transudate:** hypoalbuminaemia, fluid overload, congestive heart failure.
- **Modified transudate:** congestive heart failure, inflammatory/obstructive processes.
- **Exudate:** pyothorax, neoplasia, infectious disease, FIP.
- **Chylothorax:** idiopathic, traumatic (ruptured thoracic duct), neoplasm, torsion of the pulmonary lobe, congestive heart failure.
- **Haemorrhage:** trauma, coagulopathy, neoplasia.

Clinical signs

- Progressive and severe breathing difficulty.

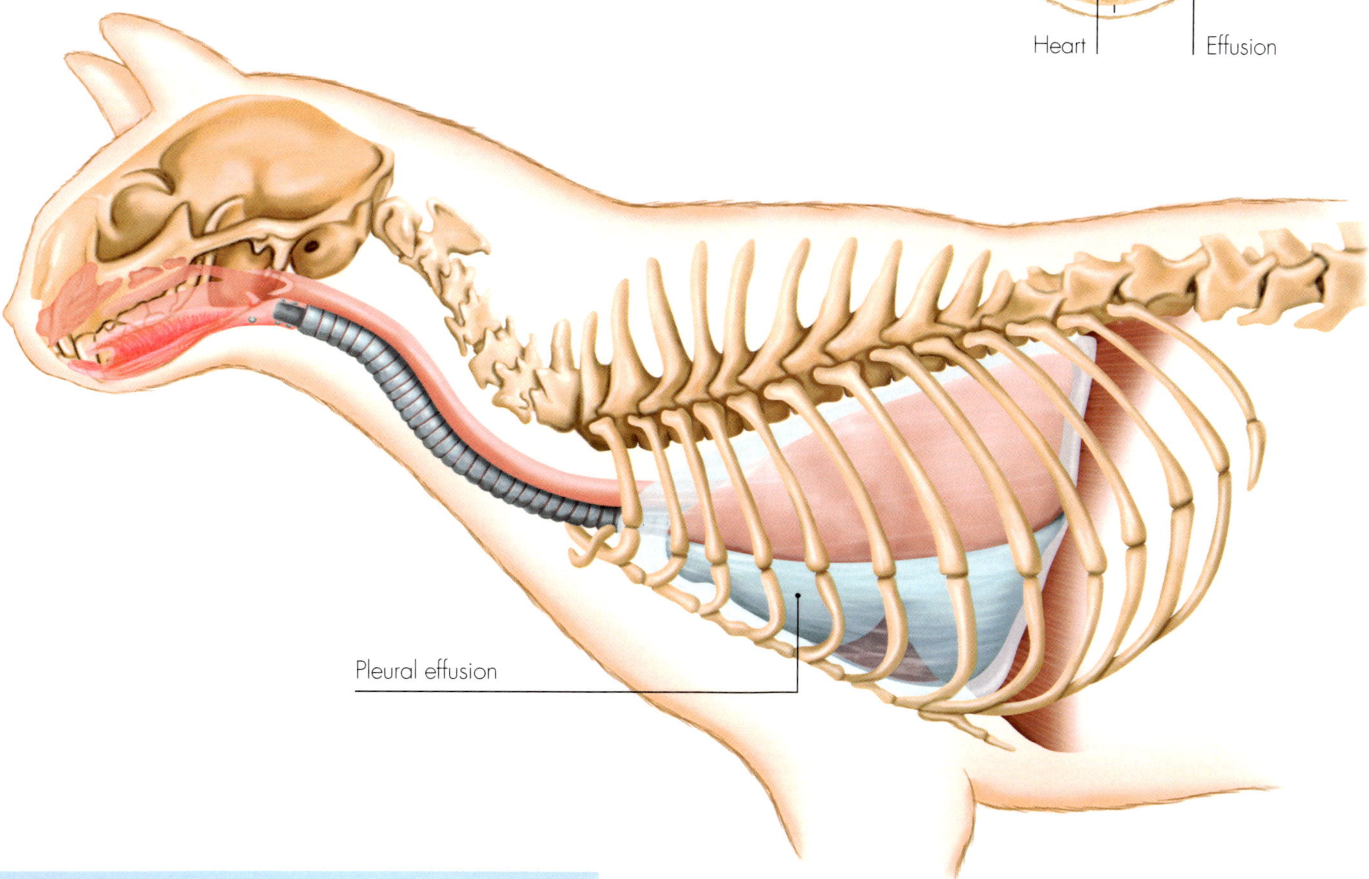

Medical/surgical treatment

It will depend on the underlying cause of the effusion.

The removal of the fluid allows the diagnosis of the cause of the pleural effusion (analysis) and the cat to breathe easily again.

CARDIORESPIRATORY SYSTEM

36 Diaphragmatic hernia

traumatic and peritoneopericardial

Traumatic

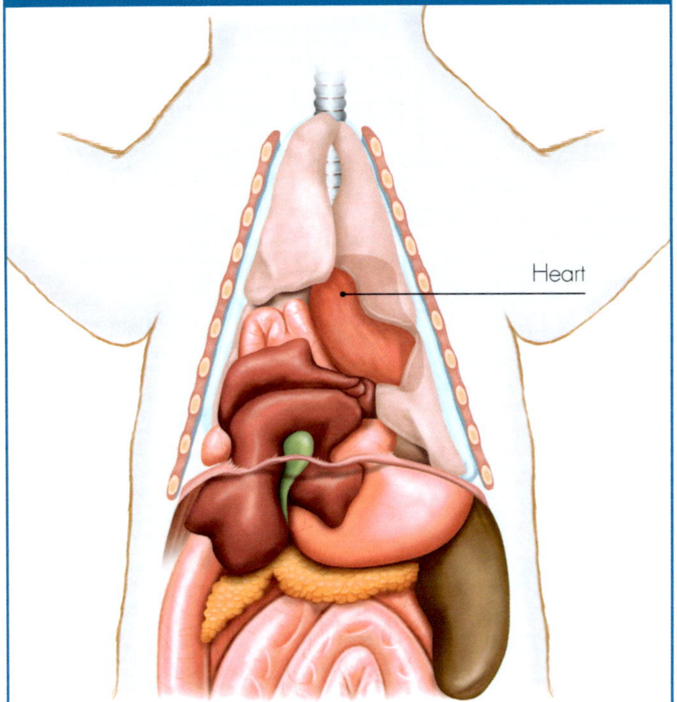

The traumatic rupture of the diaphragm allows the passage of one or various abdominal organs into the thoracic cavity.

- **Causes**: road traffic accidents or high-rise falls.
- **Clinical signs:**
  - Acute form: breathing difficulty and rib cage pain.
  - Chronic form (when it is has not been diagnosed or treated), depending on the herniated abdominal organs:
    - Difficulty breathing with exercise.
    - Depression, anorexia.
    - Digestive signs.

Peritoneopericardial

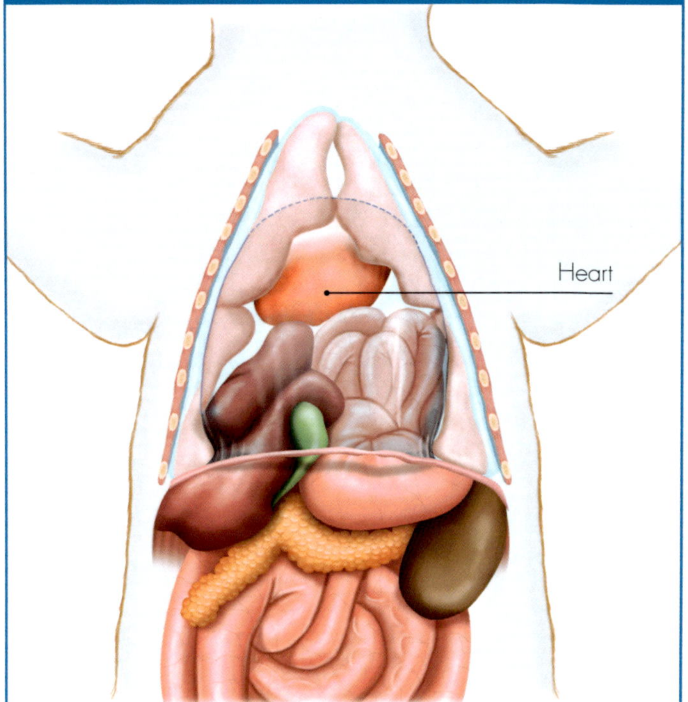

- **Causes:** congenital problem causing the pericardium and peritoneal cavity to be communicated, with the heart permanently surrounded by abdominal structures.
- **Predisposition:** long-haired cats and Himalayans.
- **Clinical signs:**
  - They depend on the herniated organ and on whether it receives appropriate blood supply. It generally affects the liver, small intestine, spleen and stomach.
  - It may be asymptomatic.
  - Gastrointestinal signs and anorexia if it affects the intestine.

Surgical treatment

- To repair the diaphragm.
- In a peritoneopericardial hernia, when it causes clinical symptoms (gastrointestinal obstruction) or when the blood flow to abdominal organs is altered.
- If a hepatic lobe or part of the abdominal fat is herniated, and there are no clinical signs, surgery may be required.

ENDOCRINE SYSTEM

37 Hyperthyroidism

Uncontrolled production of thyroid hormones, thyroxine (T_4) and triiodothyronine (T_3), by the thyroid gland, either due to nodular hyperplasia or to a benign adenoma, although 1 % of the affected animals will develop thyroid carcinoma.

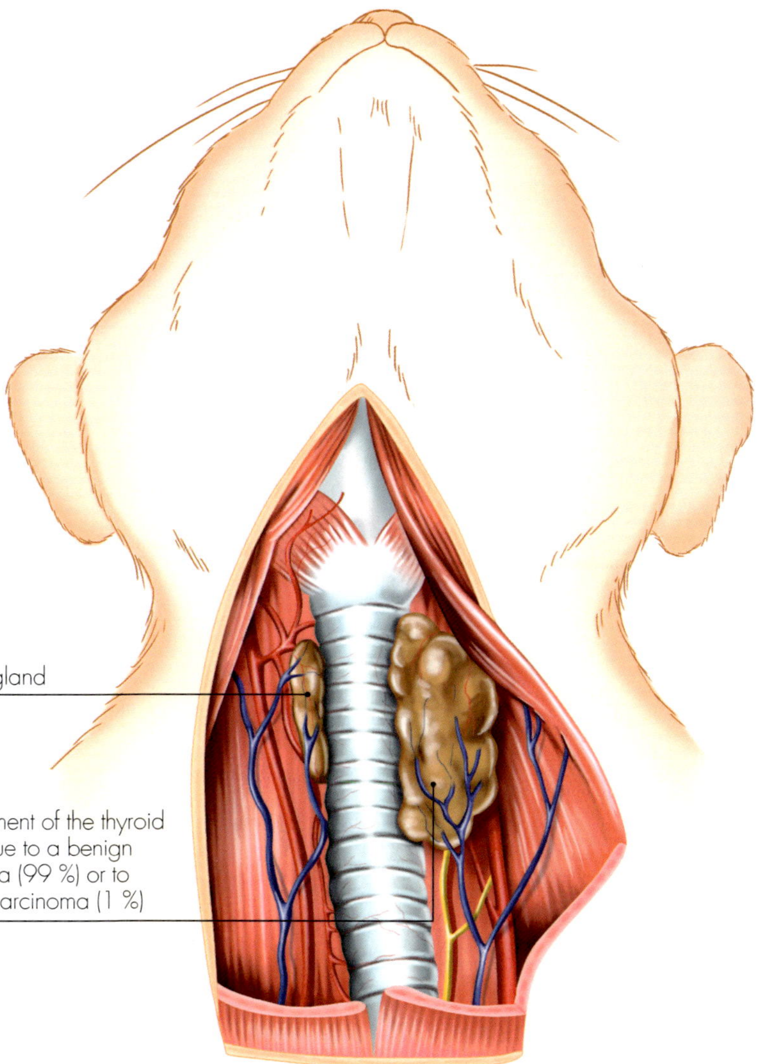

Risk factors

- Cats >6 years old.
- Goitrogenic substances present in easy-open tins and in additives contained in fish-based or liver-based wet food.
- Diets with very variable iodine concentrations (from deficient to excessive).

Clinical signs

- Unilateral or bilateral nodule in the cervical region (80–90 % of cases).
- Progressive loss of weight, polyphagia, hyperactivity.
- Digestive: chronic vomiting, diarrhoea.
- Cardiac: hypertension, hypertrophic cardiomyopathy.
- Hepatic: increased hepatic enzyme levels.

It is the most frequent endocrine disease in cats.

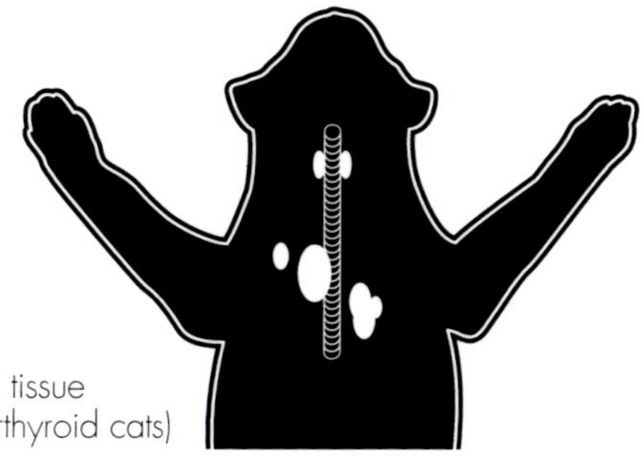

Treatment

- Chronic treatment: with oral drugs or a strict low-iodine diet. This controls the clinical signs but does not prevent tumour growth.
- Curative treatment:
  - Radioactive iodine (I-131).
  - Surgery (thyroidectomy).

ENDOCRINE SYSTEM

38 Feline diabetes

Risk factors

- Age: most diagnosed cats are >6 years old (greater incidence: 10–13 years of age).
- Breed: Burmese cats have a greater predisposition.
- Inactivity: very frequent in indoor cats.
- Obesity: it is the most important factor, especially in males.
- Infections and inflammations: periodontal disease, infections of the urinary tract, pyoderma, pancreatitis, etc.
- Treatment with corticosteroids or progestogens.

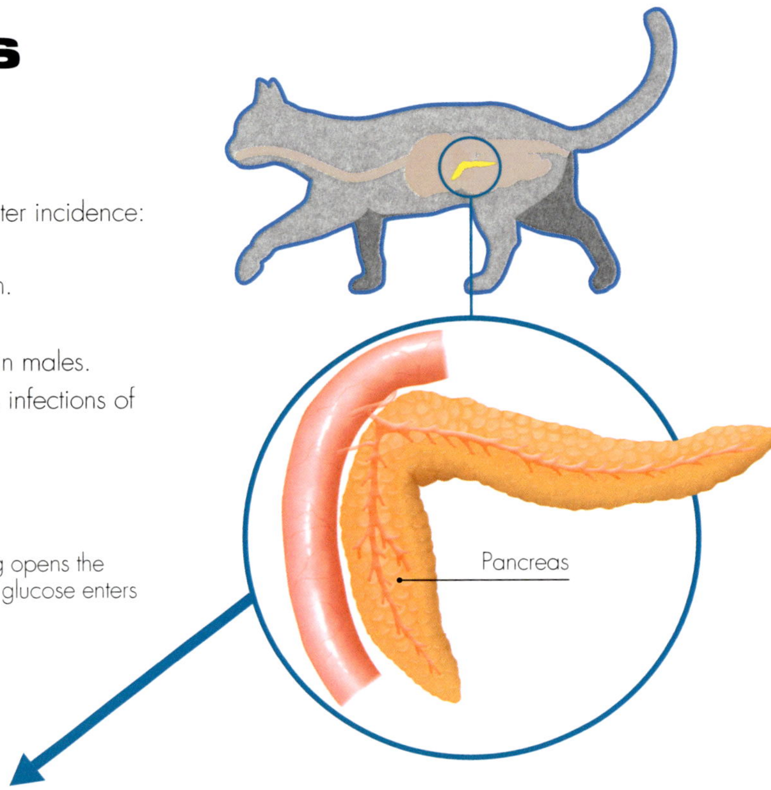

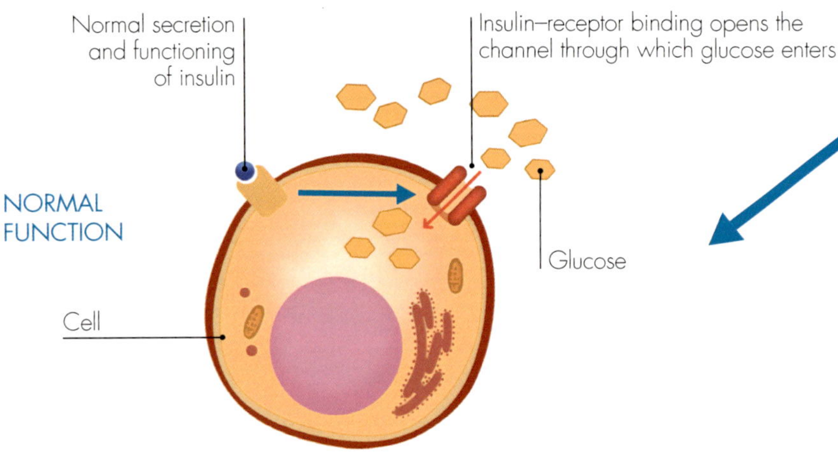

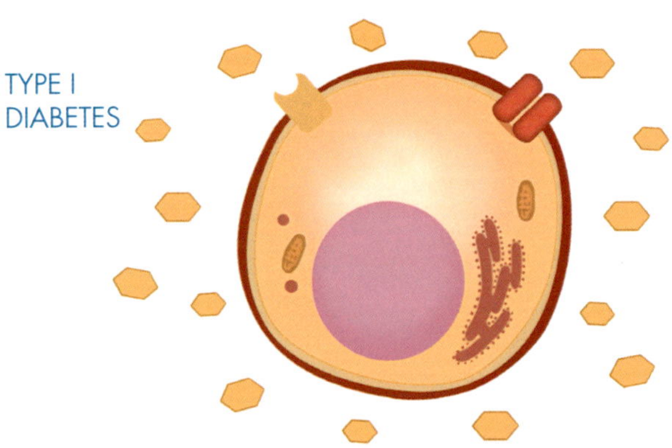

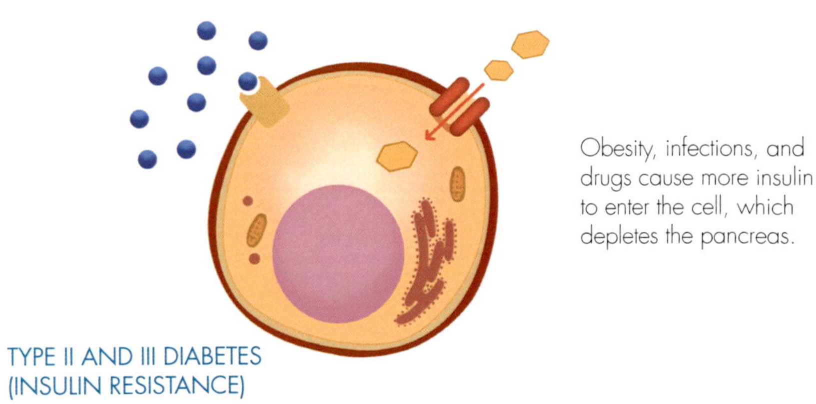

Recovery occurs in up to 67 % of the cats treated with insulin and a specific diet for diabetic cats rapidly after the diagnosis.

Clinical signs

- Polyuria/polydipsia.
- Polyphagia (they eat more).
- Loss of weight.
- Diabetic neuropathy: hind limb weakness and in acute cases, of the forelimbs too.

TYPE I DIABETES: destruction of the pancreatic cells by the immune system.

TYPE II DIABETES: combination of an inappropriate secretion of insulin and resistance to its action in tissues (due to obesity, infection, etc.).

TYPE III DIABETES: due to diseases that lead to high resistance to the action of insulin: hyperadrenocorticism, acromegaly, pancreatitis, pancreatic adenocarcinoma, administration of glycocorticoids, etc.

ENDOCRINE SYSTEM

39 Acromegaly

Acromegaly occurs when the pituitary gland produces excess growth hormone due to the presence of an adenoma or, less commonly, a carcinoma. It is the cause of type III diabetes in cats, since the excess of growth hormone means that insulin receptors are occupied and therefore become resistant to its action. For this reason, control of diabetic cats becomes increasingly complex.

Clinical signs

Clinical signs are observed in only 25 % of acromegalic cats, since it is a progressive disease and the onset of diabetes precedes the appearance of clinical signs of acromegaly:

- Prognathism (protrusion of the jaw) (18 %).
- Increase in face size (37 %).
- Weight gain.
- Increase in the size of the abdominal organs (40 %).
- Increased limb size (13 %).

Diagnosis

- Measurement of IGF-1* concentration in all diabetic cats after weeks of insulin treatment. An IGF-1 value >1,000 ng/ml has a positive predictive value of 95 %.
- Computed tomography (CT) confirms the diagnosis when an increase in the size of the pituitary gland is observed.
- Magnetic resonance imaging (MRI) can diagnose cases for which the CT scan is negative.

Normal cat

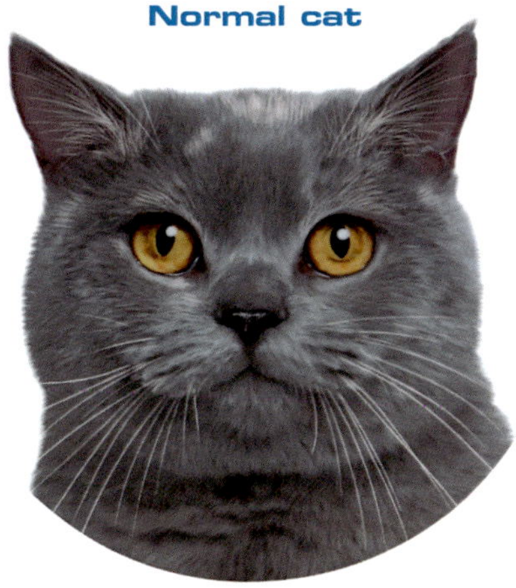

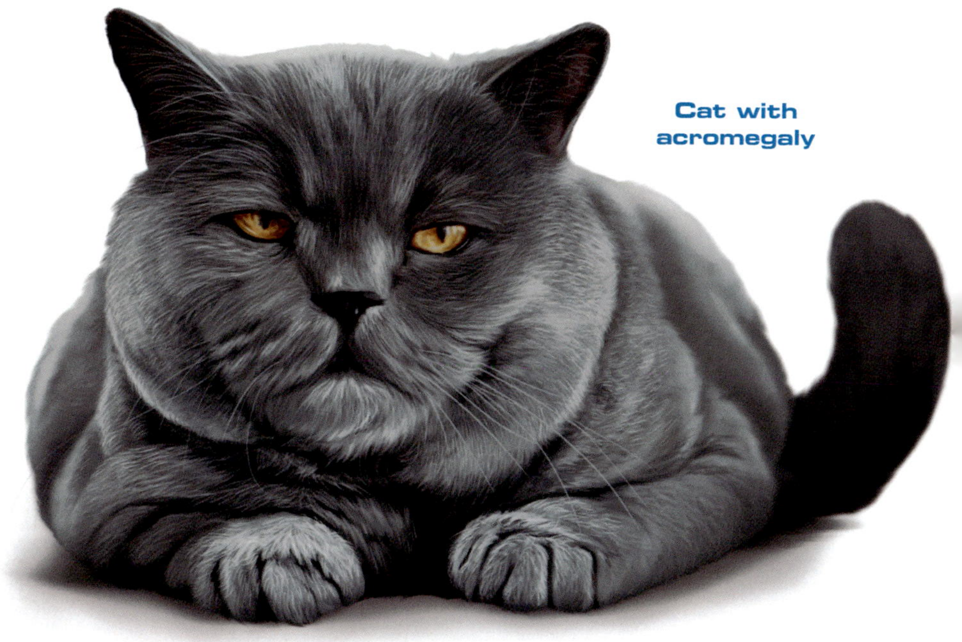

Cat with acromegaly

One in four diabetic cats may have acromegaly.

Treatment

- Medical: pasireotide appears to reduce hormone levels and improve diabetes management.
- Radiotherapy: reduces the size of the pituitary gland and allows better control of diabetes.
- Surgery: removal of the pituitary (this is a very complex surgical technique).

* IGF-1: somatomedin C or insulin-like growth factor 1.

ENDOCRINE SYSTEM

40 Obesity

Obesity is a serious disease that must be treated with diet and lifestyle changes.

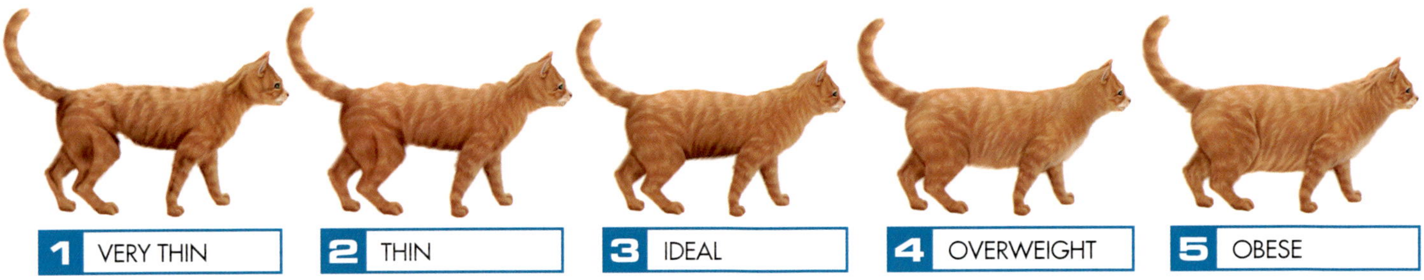

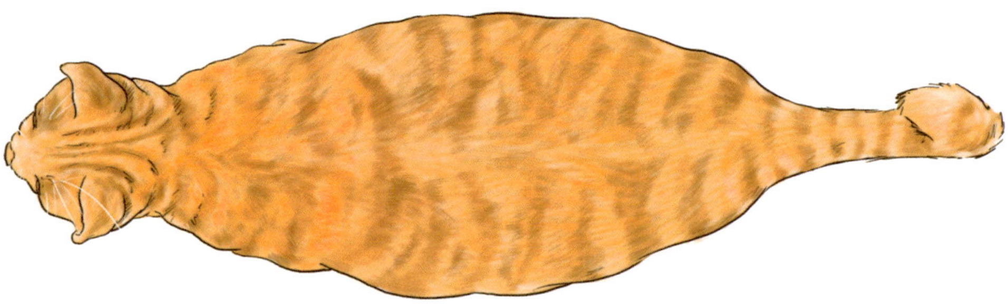

Risk factors

- Neutering: it reduces the energy needs of cats by 20 %.
- Inactivity: frequent in indoor cats.
- Age: cats between 2 and 10 years old are the most prone to it.
- Feeding: food with a high calorie content and great palatability.

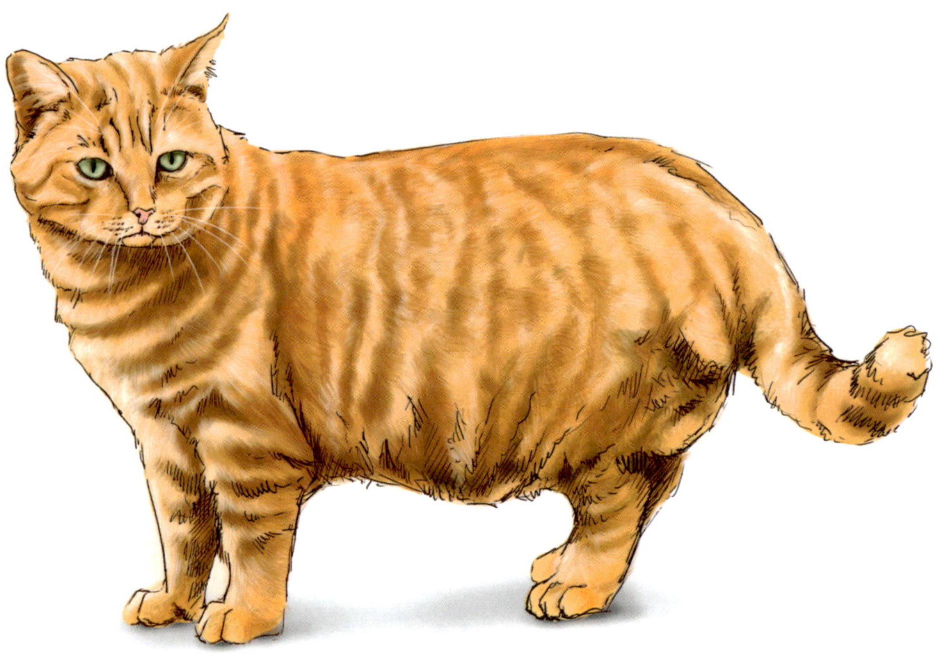

Obesity increases the risk of suffering from certain diseases.

Associated complications

- Diabetes mellitus.
- Osteoarthritis.
- Hepatic lipidosis.
- Skin alterations.
- Respiratory problems.
- Dystocia.
- Intolerance to exercise.
- Lower immune functions.
- Greater anaesthetic risk.
- Shorter life expectancy.

Recommendations

Increased daily activity by means of interactive food dispensers and increased daily play (*Nepeta cataria* plant –catnip–, laser pointers, etc.).

Dietary treatment

Calorie-restricted diets.

SKIN AND ANEXA

41 Structures of the skin in cats

Skin layers

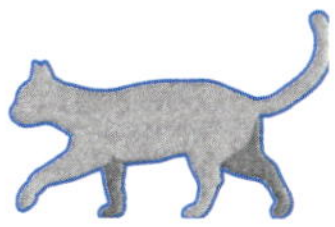

1. Epidermis.
2. Dermis.
3. Subcutaneous tissue or hypodermis.

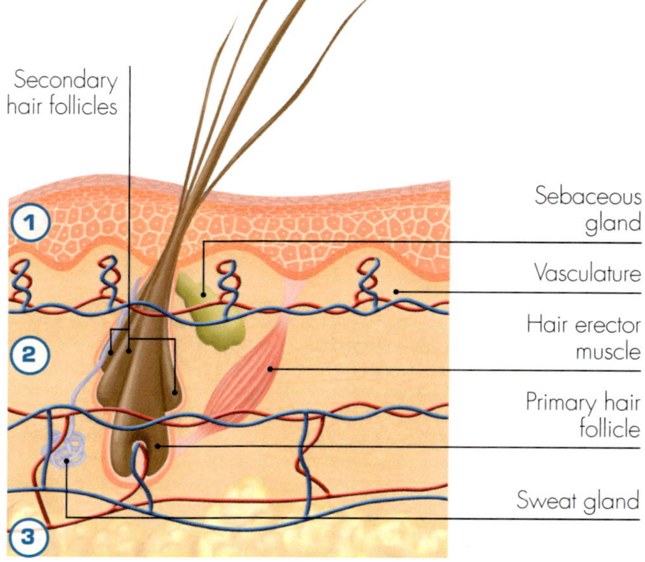

NORMAL HAIR

Hair grows to a certain length, which varies depending on the body region and is genetically predetermined.

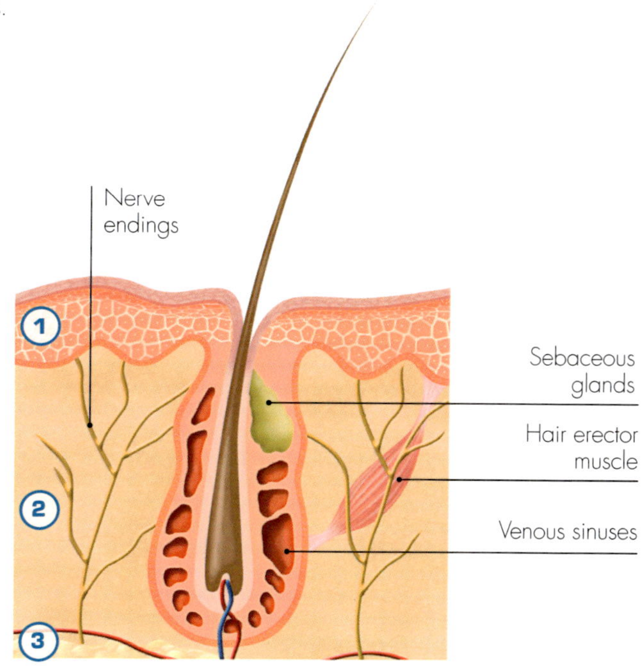

TACTILE HAIR OR VIBRISSA

- They are located on each side of their nose, above their eyes, below their ears (angle of the mandible) and at the back of their carpus.
- They are very sensitive to pressure or to air currents.

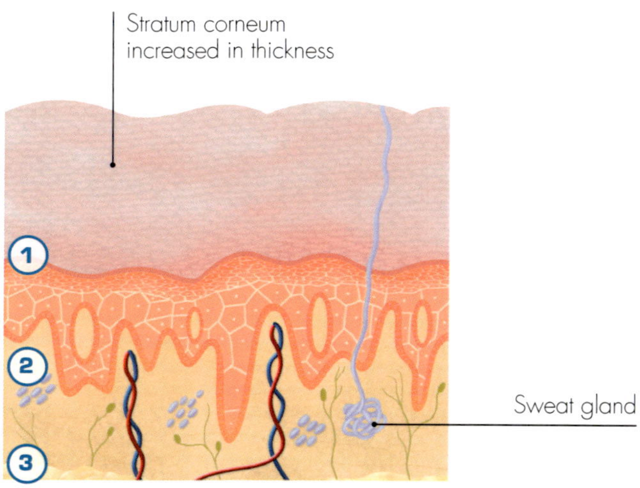

FOOTPAD

- Protective tissue of the paws that also provides cushioning.
- They secrete pheromones through sweat.

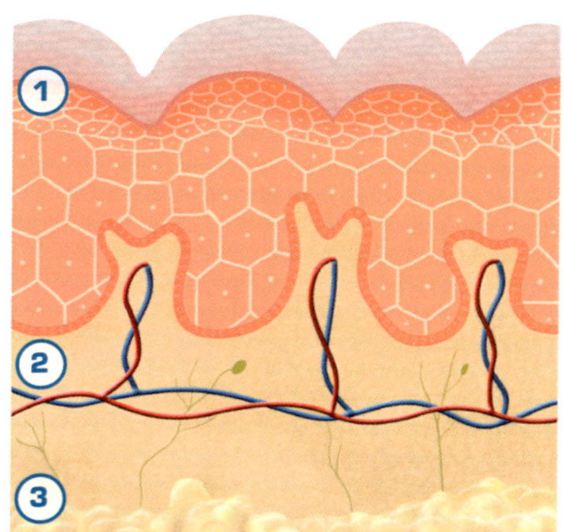

NASAL EPITHELIUM

- It may have different colours depending on the cat's breed and coat.
- Its temperature and degree of humidity are not always an indication of the cat's state of health.

SKIN AND ANEXA

42 Characteristics of claws

Disorders of claws

- Macronychia: abnormally long claws.
- Onychalgia: pain in the claws.
- Onychoclasis: breaking of claws.
- Onychocryptosis (onyxis): ingrown claws.
- Onychodystrophy: abnormal claw formation.
- Onychogryphosis: hypertrophy and abnormal curvature of claws.
- Onychomadesis: sloughing of claws.
- Onychomalacia: softening of claws.
- Onychorrhexis: longitudinal striations and breaking of claws.
- Onychoschizia: splitting or lamination of claws.
- Onychia (onychitis): inflammation of part of the claw.
- Paronychia: inflammation/infection of the folds of tissue surrounding the claw.

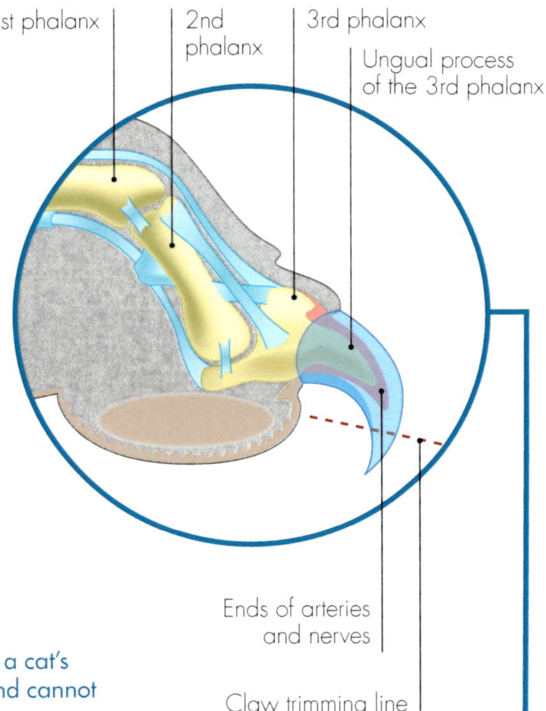

Scratching is part of a cat's natural behaviour and cannot be eliminated.

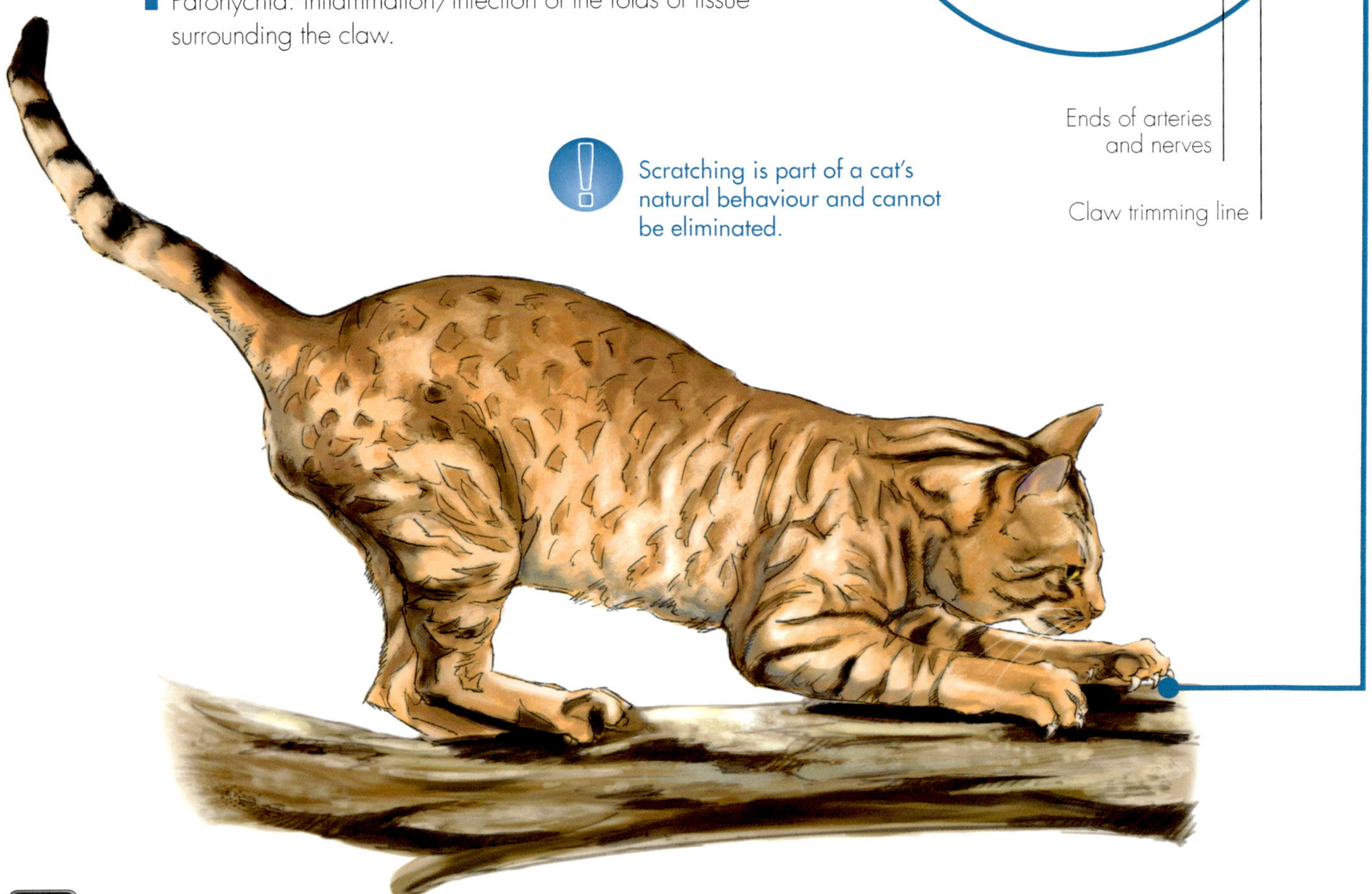

Recommendations

To prevent a cat form scratching sofas or other furniture, the following should be done:

- Place a scratcher in the area where the cat usually rests.
- Scratchers should be sturdy and not wobble when scratched. Scratching posts are ideal.
- If the cat already scratches a sofa or other surface, this latter should be cleaned and an adequate scratching post should be placed next to it.
- A cat should not be forced to use a scratcher. Instead, play should be used to encourage the cat to scratch it.

SKIN AND ANEXA

43 Feline acne

An increase in the activity of the sebaceous glands in the chin leads to the formation of blackheads, which are particularly noticeable in pale-coloured cats.

The diagnostic tests are: cutaneous cytology, skin scraping, biopsy and bacterial and fungal cultures.

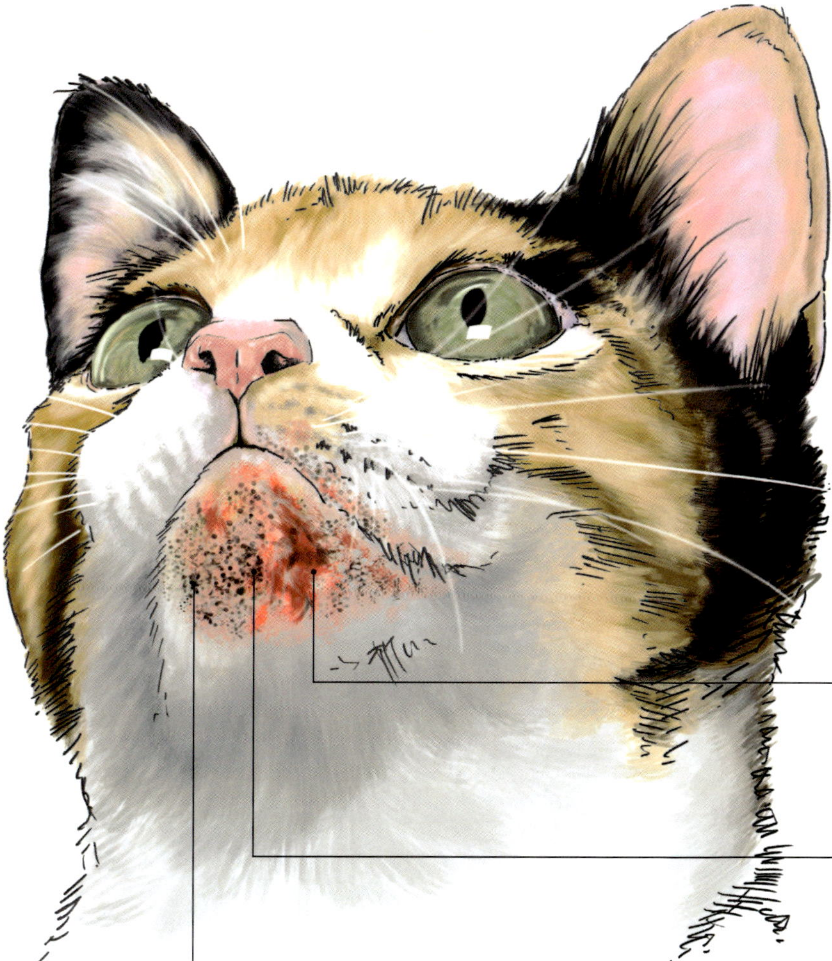

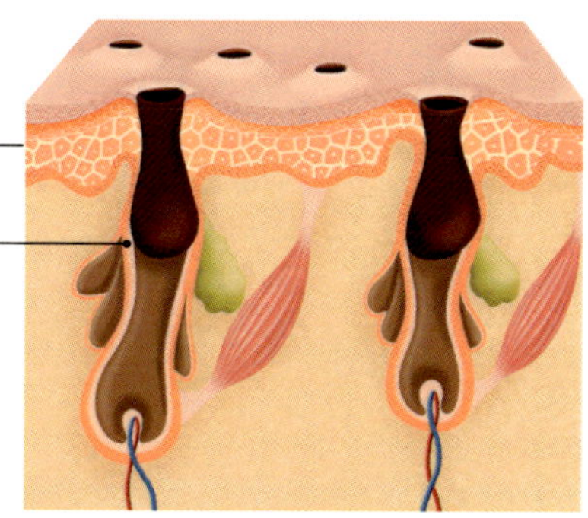

Triggering factors

Multifactorial process:

- Greater production of fat.
- Immunosuppression and stress.
- Respiratory viruses (whether they are direct causative agents or responsible for immunosuppresion and stress is under research).
- Bacterial overgrowth.

Medical treatment

Depending on the severity, the administration of a combination of drugs (antibiotics, antifungal medication, corticosteroids, essential fatty acids, etc.) by oral and topical routes will be required.

Clinical signs

- Blackheads on the chin, upper lip and labial commissure.
- If it worsens, erythema, pustules and even firm and inflamed nodules (furunculosis) will appear. Abscesses in very severe cases.
- Itching in case of bacterial infection.

SKIN AND ANEXA

44 Feline hypersensitivity

Allergies

Hypersensitivity is an excessive and inappropriate immune response to usually harmless allergens. It leads to skin and sometimes digestive disorders.

Clinical signs

Itching associated with one or various patterns of reaction:

- Symmetrical alopecia.
- Miliary dermatitis.
- Eosinophilic granuloma complex.
- Pruritus on the face and neck.

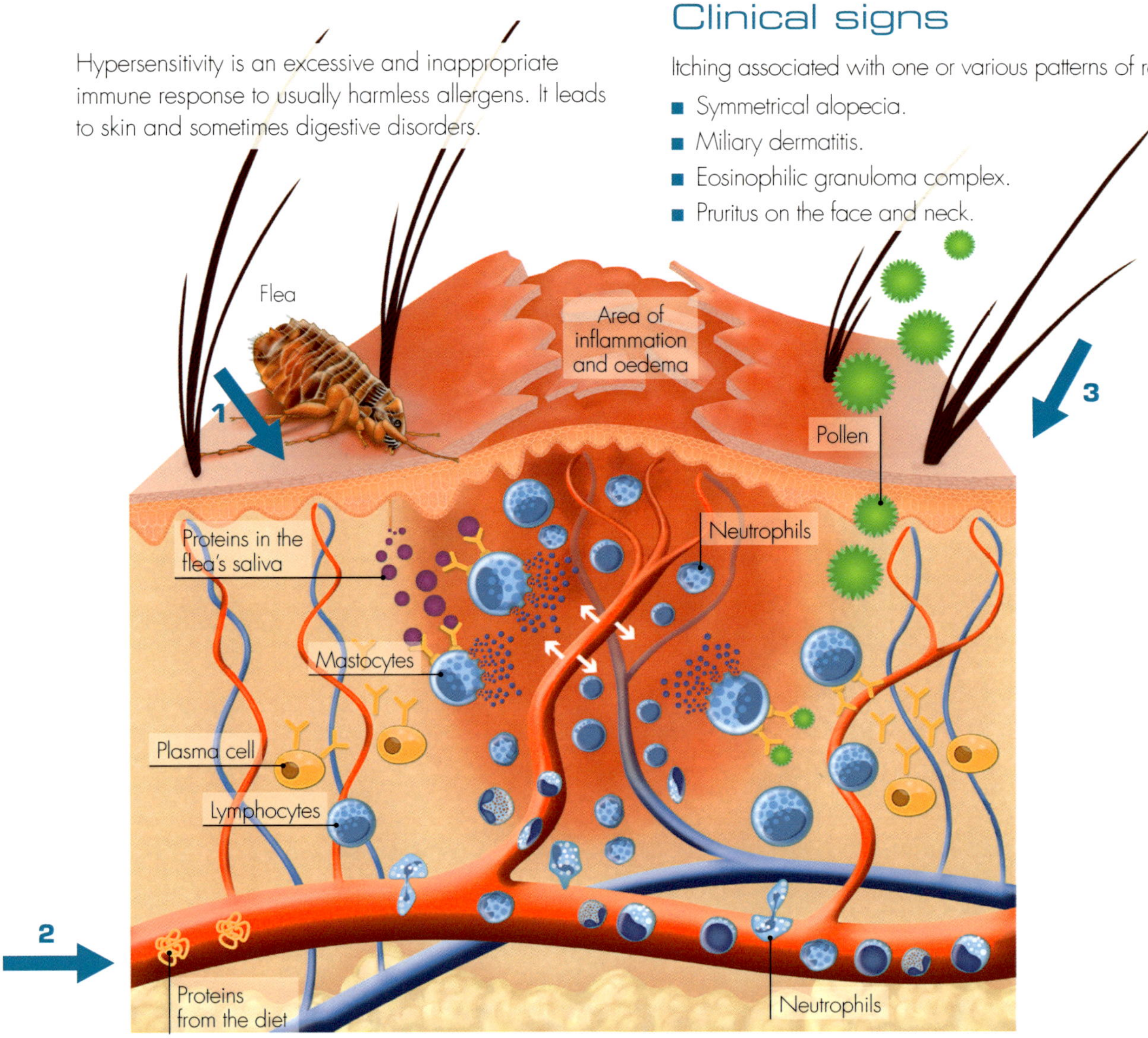

1 Hypersensitivity to flea bites

- Fleas release substances that cause inflammatory reactions at the bite site.
- It is the first cause of hypersensitivity to rule out.
- Treatment: adulticides together with products to control larvae and eggs in the environment.

2 Adverse reaction to food

- Cats between 3 months and 12 years of age.
- Cutaneous and/or digestive clinical signs. Less frequent: interdigital erythema, acne, pododermatitis, conjunctivitis and angioedema.
- Allergens: fish, dairy products, beef, chicken, lamb, gluten, additives, corn and rice.
- Treatment: diet excluding the foods the cat is allergic to.

3 Atopic dermatitis

- Cats between 6 months and 3 years of age.
- Otitis, pododermatitis and seborrheic alterations may be observed together with pruritus and the aforementioned patterns of reaction.
- Allergens: dust mites and pollens.
- Treatment: immunotherapy with hyposensitisation vaccines (70–80 % efficacy).

SKIN AND ANEXA

45 Feline eosinophilic granuloma complex

The eosinophilic granuloma complex is a cutaneous reaction pattern caused by hypersensitivity (atopy, adverse reaction to food, hypersensitivity to flea bites). It has three manifestations: indolent ulcer, eosinophilic granuloma and eosinophilic plaque.

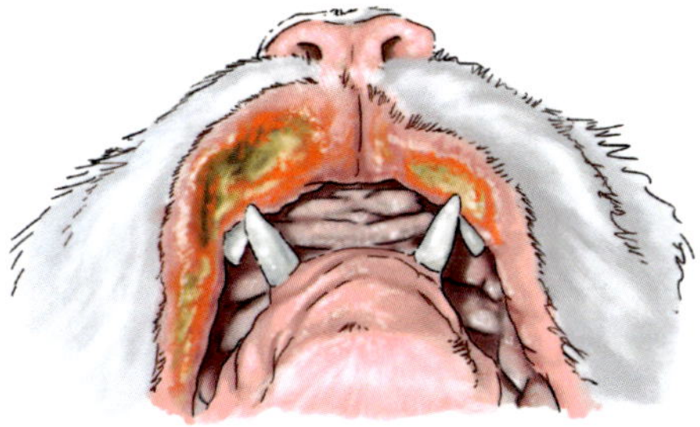

Indolent ulcer

- Ulcerative lesion of the upper lip which can extend to the hard palate.
- It may be uni- or bilateral and, in spite of its appearance, it does not cause pain.

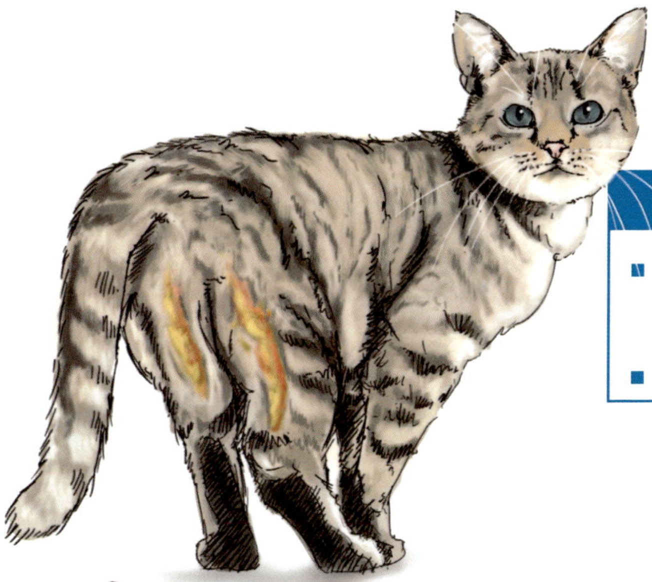

Linear granuloma

- Yellowish to pink linear lesions on the back of one or the two hind legs. It may also appear in the oral cavity, forelimbs and chin (chin oedema).
- There is no associated pruritus or pain.

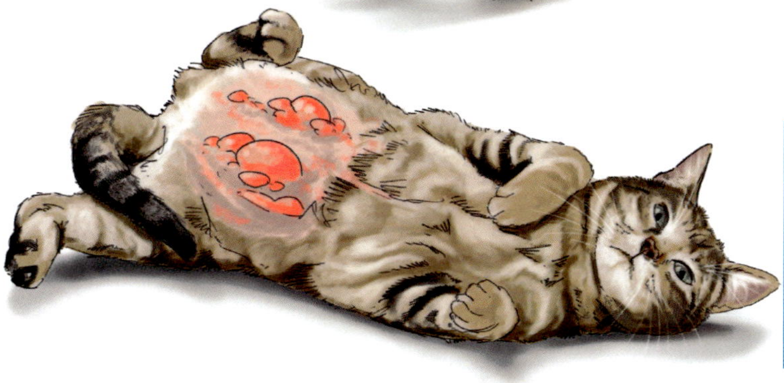

Eosinophilic plaque

- Erythematous (reddish) and ulcerated lesions in the form of a plaque and located on the abdomen, inner thighs, inguinal region, neck and interdigital spaces.
- Pruritus is severe.

Medical treatment

The definitive treatment involves the diagnosis of the cat's hypersensitivity.

SKIN AND ANEXA

46 Alopecia

The new clinical approach to alopecia is to first observe its distribution pattern and then the lesions that accompany the alopecia.

Clinical approach to alopecia according to distribution patterns			
Focal o multifocal	Irregular	Regional	Generalised
■ Demodicosis ■ Superficial pyoderma ■ Dermatophytosis ■ Alopecia areata ■ Cutaneous asthenia ■ Traction alopecia ■ Inflammatory reaction at the site of injection ■ Cicatricial alopecia	■ Demodicosis ■ Cheyletiellosis ■ Dermatophytosis ■ Pediculosis ■ Rash caused by drugs ■ Lupus erythematosus ■ Telogen effluvium ■ Hyperadrenocorticism	■ Lupus erythematosus ■ Endocrine alopecia ■ Hyperadrenocorticism ■ Psychogenic alopecia ■ Post-clipping alopecia ■ Alopecia of the ears ■ Acquired symmetrical alopecia ■ Paraneoplastic alopecia	■ Dermatophytosis ■ Lupus erythematosus ■ Reaction to drugs ■ Alopecia areata ■ Hypotrichosis ■ Telogen effluvium
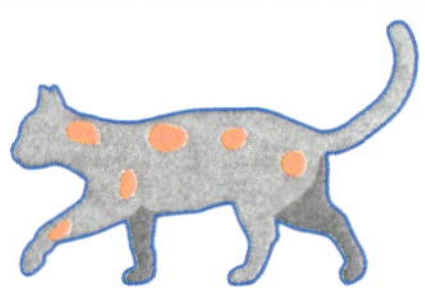	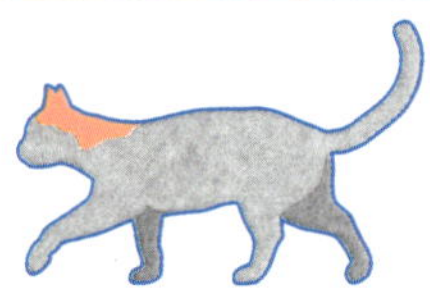	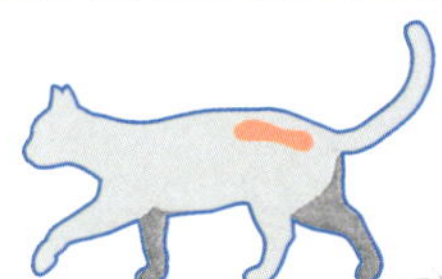	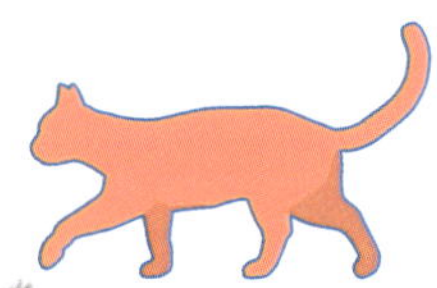

In addition to the focal, multifocal, irregular, regional or generalised absence of hair, alopecia may be accompanied, depending on the cause, by other secondary clinical signs such as pruritus, inflammation, scabs, scaling, pustules, etc.

Diagnosis

- Several tests may be necessary to determine the cause of the alopecia and apply the specific treatment.
- Usual tests: skin scrapings, trichograms, fungal cultures, skin biopsies, blood tests and determination of hormone levels.

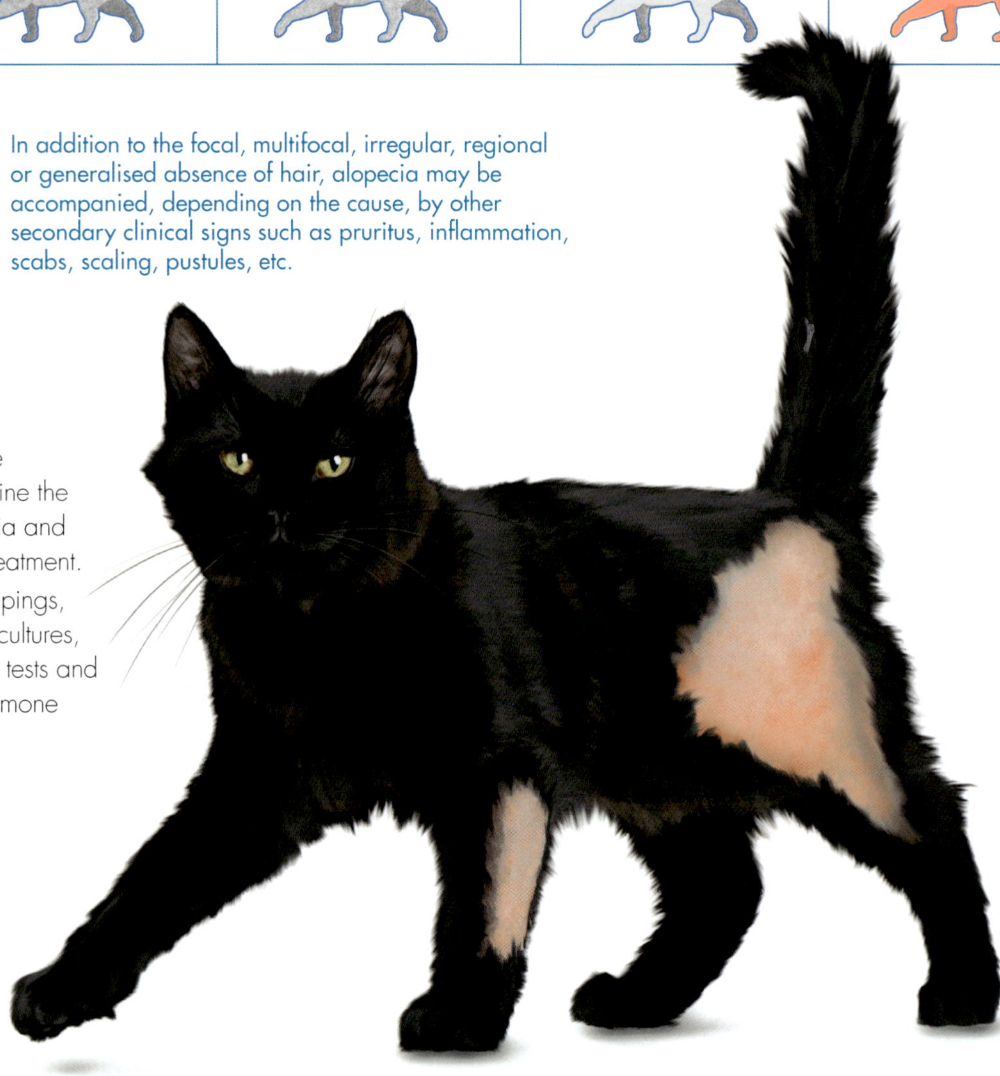

SKIN AND ANEXA

47 Idiopathic facial dermatitis in Persian and Himalayan cats

While its origin is unknown, this can be a hereditary disease. It manifests as an abnormally abundant seborrheic discharge, which favours the proliferation of bacteria and yeasts (*Malasezzia*). It usually occurs in cats between 10 months and 6 years of age and must be differentiated from other conditions such as demodicosis, feline acne, dermatophytosis and hypersensitivity.

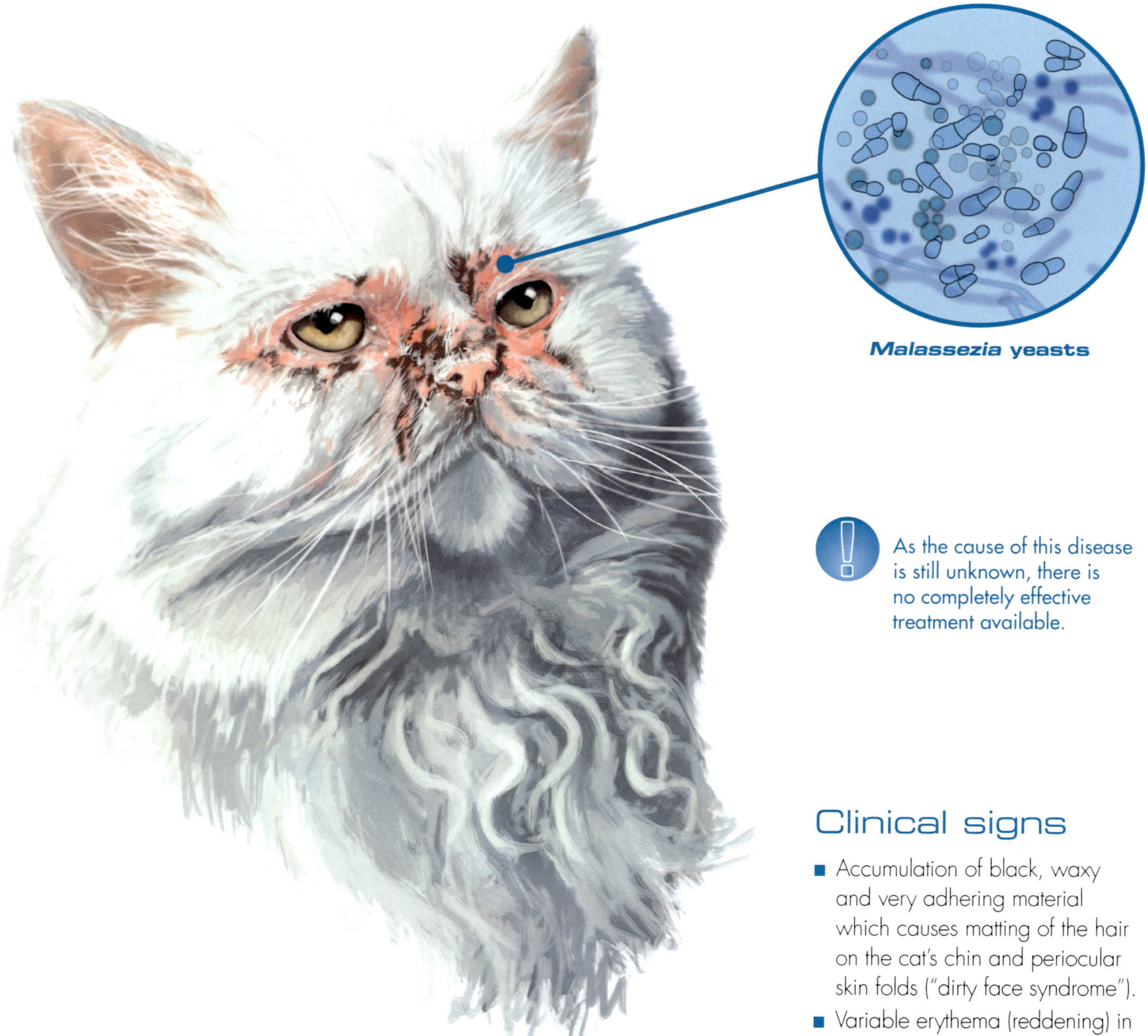

***Malassezia* yeasts**

As the cause of this disease is still unknown, there is no completely effective treatment available.

Clinical signs

- Accumulation of black, waxy and very adhering material which causes matting of the hair on the cat's chin and periocular skin folds ("dirty face syndrome").
- Variable erythema (reddening) in the affected regions.
- In many cases, bilateral erythematous dermatitis.
- Complication with the growth of bacteria and *Malassezia*.
- Submandibular lymphadenopathy (occasionally).

Medical treatment

- It focuses on controlling infections caused by bacteria and yeasts with oral products and topical lotions.
- After achieving control of the infection, treatment with prednisolone or cyclosporine can be successful in some cats.

SKIN AND ANEXA

48 Dermatophytosis

It is an infection of the skin, hair and claws caused by the fungi *Microsporum*, *Trochophyton* and *Epidermophyton*.

Disease transmissible to humans (zoonosis).

A cat is not considered cured until at least two negative cultures at a 2-week interval have been obtained. If the results are positive, the medical treatment should be maintained.

Clinical signs

- Focal alopecia, with round lesions on the head, face, and forelimbs.
- Localised lesions that may become generalised.
- Scaling.
- Variable degrees of itching, from non-existent to intense.
- Variable degrees of inflammation.

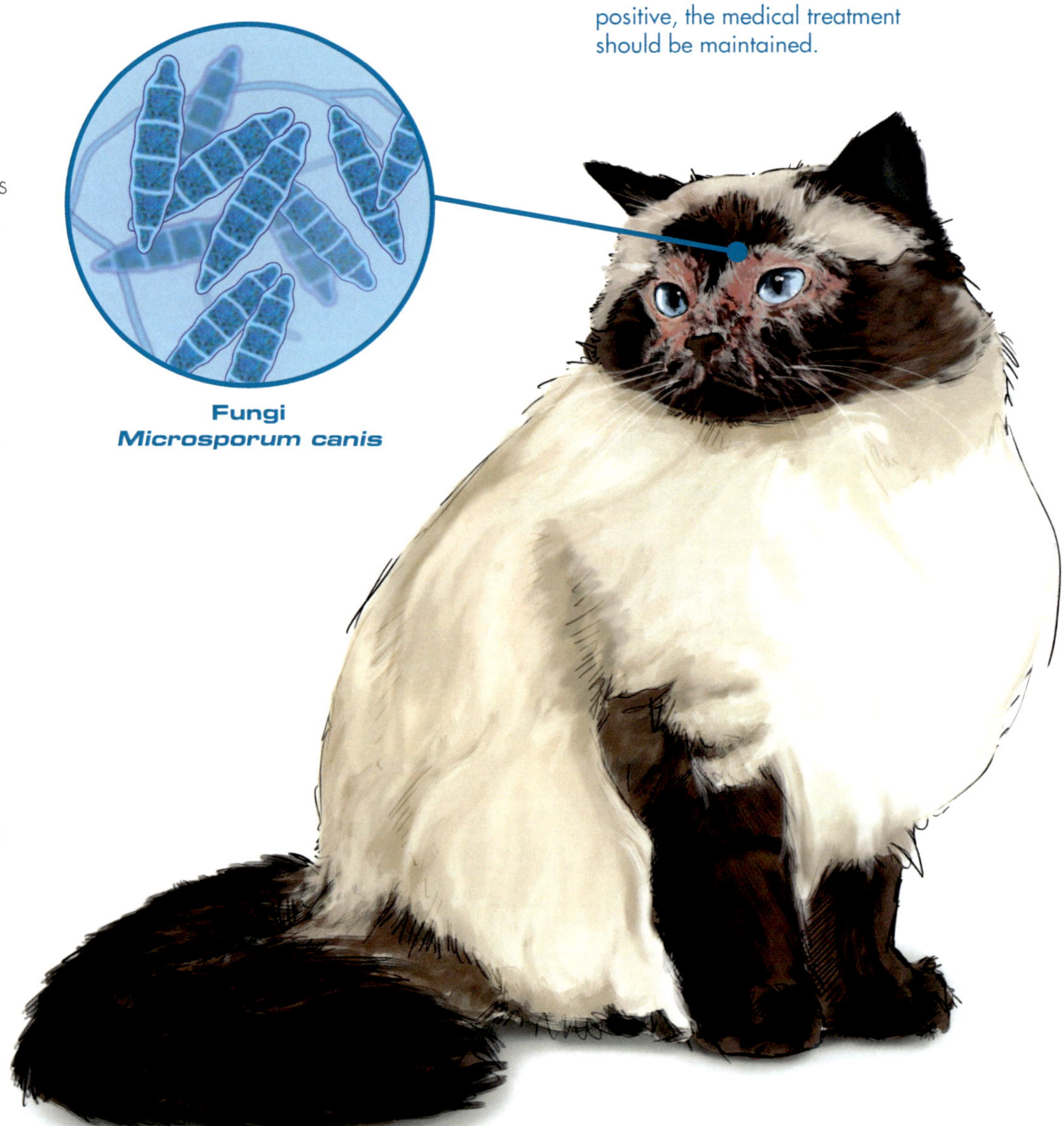

Fungi
Microsporum canis

Predisposing factors

- Cats <1 year of age.
- Long hair.
- Cats living in groups.
- Immunosuppression.
- Cutaneous trauma, poor aeration or excessive humidity of the skin.

Medical treatment

- Topical: shampoo 2 times/week (reduces environmental contamination).
- Hair clipping 2–3 weeks after starting the oral treatment (reduces environmental contamination and possible reinfections).
- Oral (systemic) treatment with itraconazole.

Recommendations

- Disinfection of the environment: vacuum clean every day and change the bag frequently.
- Fungicide products are of limited use due to the difficulty in applying them everywhere in the household.

SKIN AND ANEXA

49 Feline notoedric mange

It is caused by the mite *Notoedres cati*. It may affect other animals and people, although it is uncommon.

Notoedres cati burrows into the skin of the cat's face, head and neck to lay its eggs. Mites only survive 48 hours in the environment.

The diagnosis is made by skin scrapings.

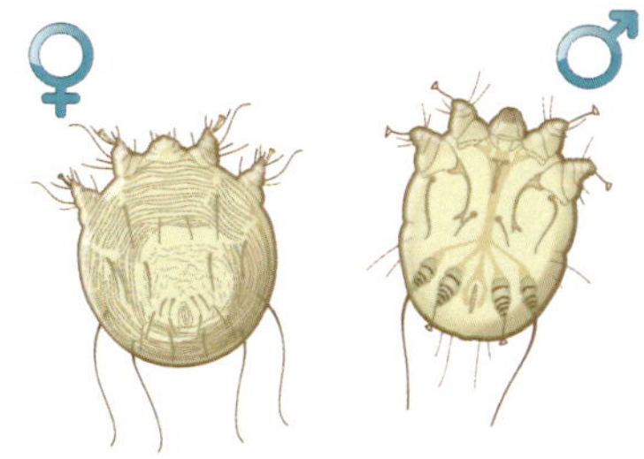

Notoedres cati mites

Young or debilitated cats are the most affected.

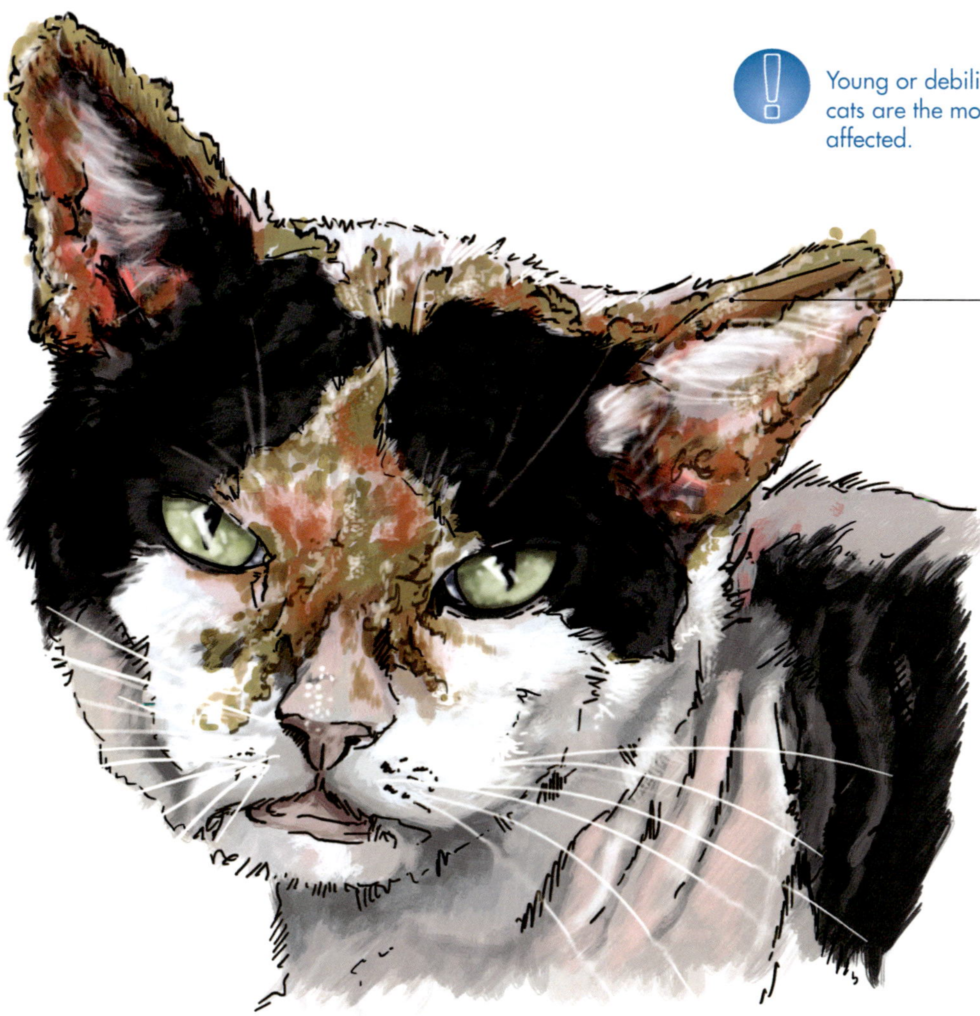

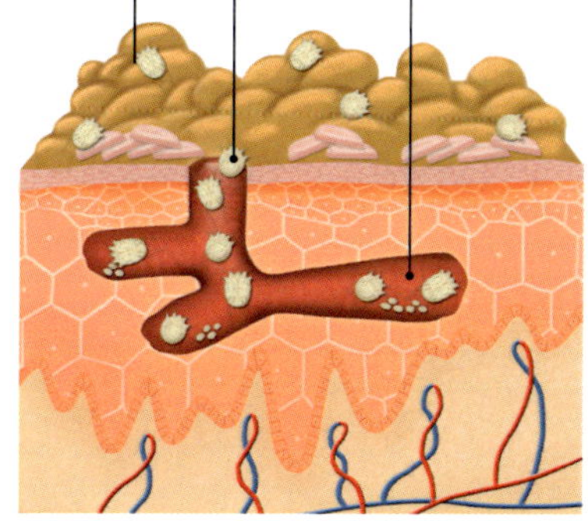

Clinical signs

- Lesions at the tip of the ears, which later extend to the face, head and neck.
- The skin is thickened and covered in scabs.
- Very intense itching; the lesions caused by scratching may become infected.
- Grooming may lead to mites extending to the perineal region and limbs.

Medical treatment

- Requires the use of antiparasitic drugs such as selamectin, moxidectin, fluralaner or sarolaner.
- All the animals in contact with the affected cat must be treated.

SKIN AND ANEXA

50 Otitis caused by *Otodectes cynotis*

The mite *Otodectes cynotis* lives mainly in the ear canal and pinna.

It is highly contagious to other cats through direct contact with infected cats or contaminated environments.

All cats living in same household or shelter, boarding kennel, etc. should be treated at the same time.

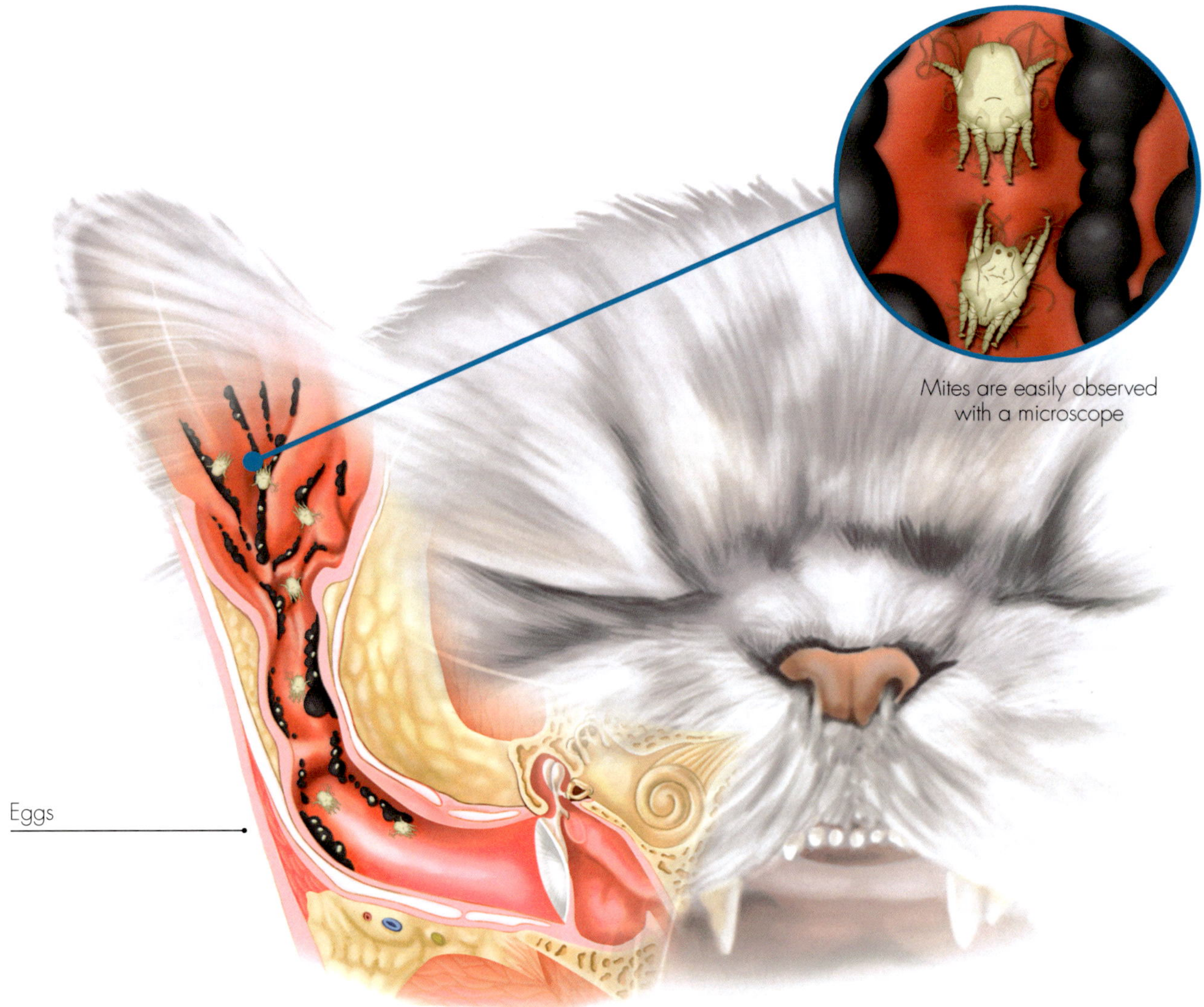

Clinical signs

- Bilateral ceruminous otitis externa.
- Reactions of hypersensitivity with intense itching, lesions caused by scratching and secondary bacterial infections.
- In severe cases, it may cause otitis media.
- Occasionally, lesions on the face and at the tip of the tail.
- Occasional miliary dermatitis.

Medical treatment

- Ear cleaning.
- Administration of a single dose of topical anti-parasitic to the skin (usually between the shoulders): selamectin, moxidectin, fluralaner, and sarolaner are effective.

SKIN AND ANEXA

51 Cutaneous tumours

Squamous cell carcinoma and fibrosarcoma

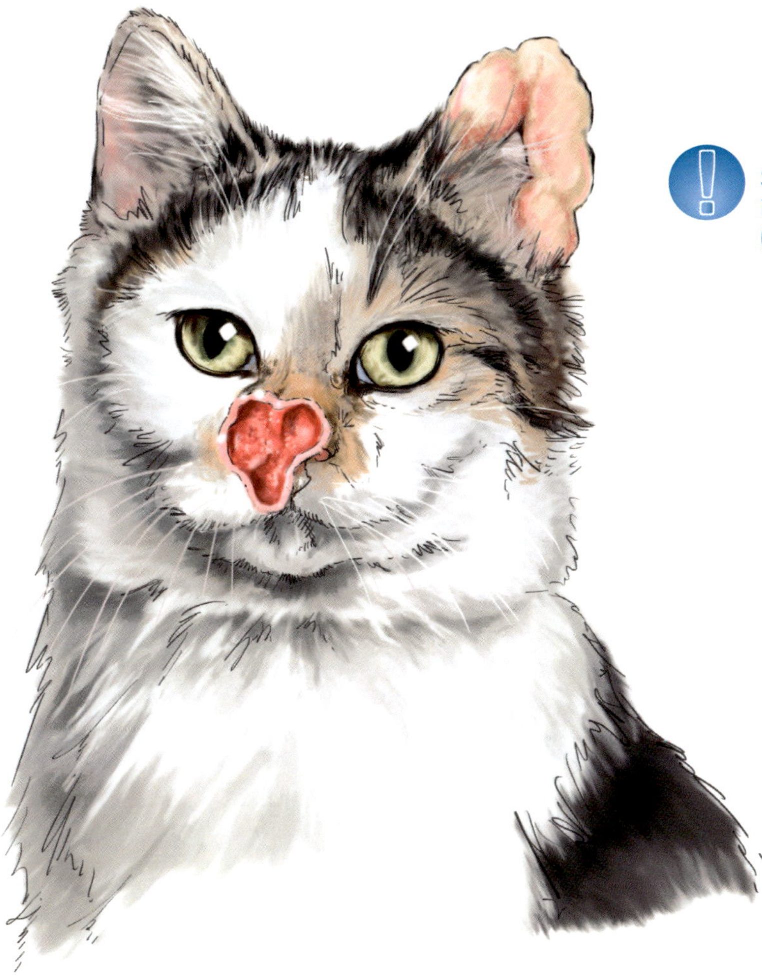

Sun protection is very important in white-haired cats (sun screen, tattooing).

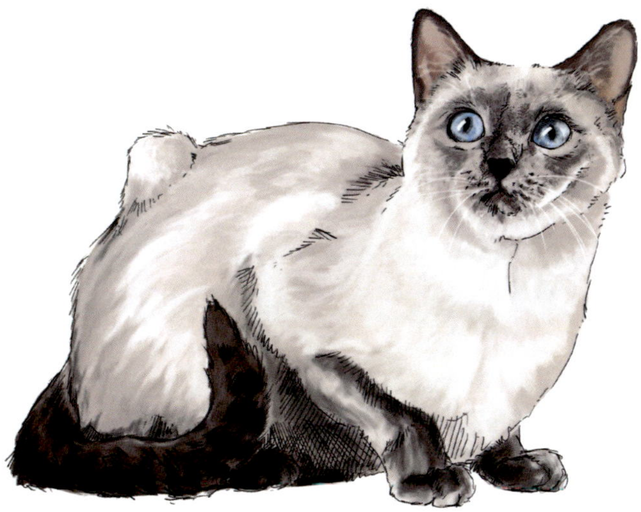

Injection-site fibrosarcoma is caused by an abnormal reaction to chronic inflammation in the tissues of some cats.

Cutaneous squamous cell carcinoma

- It occurs on the nasal plane, eyelids and tip of the ears.
- It is related to prolonged exposure to the sun in pale-coloured cats or in areas with no hair.
- Scabs and ulcerated plaques appear.
- Treatment: surgery, radiotherapy or immunomodulatory therapy depending on the extension and severity.

Fibrosarcoma (injection-site sarcoma)

- It occurs at the site of injection of vaccines, drugs (long-lasting antibiotics, corticosteroids) and other products (non-absorbable sutures, microchip).
- The tumour appears between 1 month and 10 years after the injection.
- It is fast-growing and forms firm and hard nodules.
- Treatment: surgical treatment together with chemotherapy and radiotherapy depending on the extension.

SKIN AND ANEXA

52 Ectoparasites in cats

FLEAS

- Most frequent external parasite in cats.
- They frequently cause allergic dermatitis due to the injection of saliva into their host.
- They can transmit diseases such as feline infectious anaemia.
- They live permanently on the cat.
- A single female can lay up to 50 eggs a day.
- Their eggs fall onto the floor and become larvae, pupae and adult fleas.

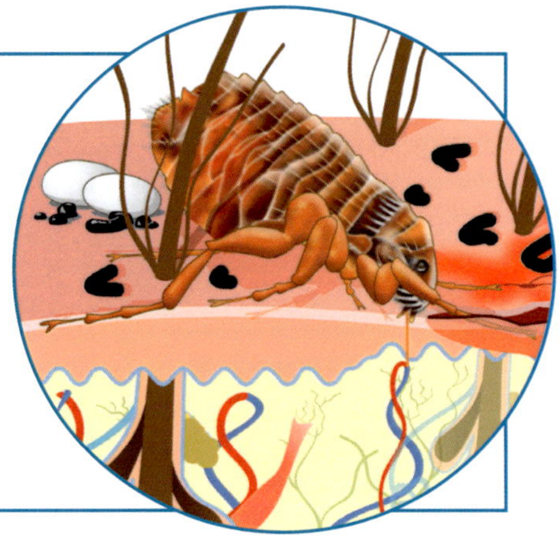

The antiparasitic control of fleas must be carried out both on the cat and on the environment.

TICKS

- They are usually of the genus *Rhipicephalus* (dog tick).
- They may cause local irritation as they inject toxins into their host.
- They transmit diseases (ehrlichiosis, Lyme disease and babesiosis).

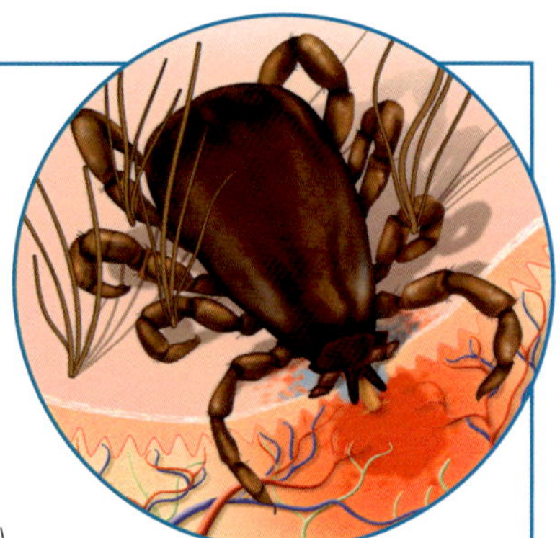

MOSQUITOES

- They bite in areas with less hair: ear margins, on the nose and on the footpads.
- They frequently cause allergic dermatitis.
- They transmit leishmaniasis and filariasis.

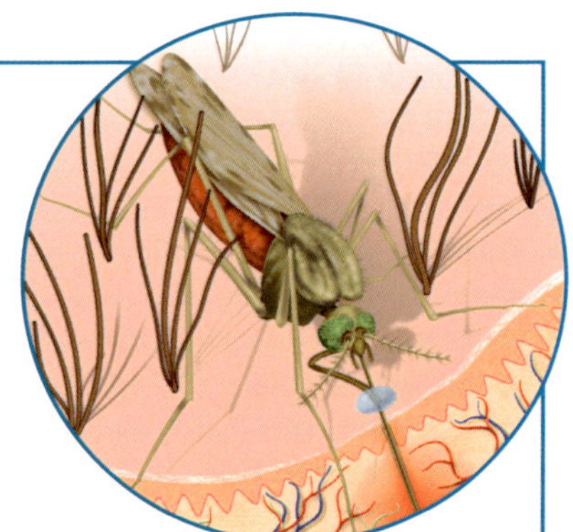

MITES*

- *Demodex cati:* demodectic mange is uncommon in cats. It causes from very mild clinical signs to severe skin disease.
- *Cheyletiella:* is a large and whitish mite, and therefore looks like dandruff.

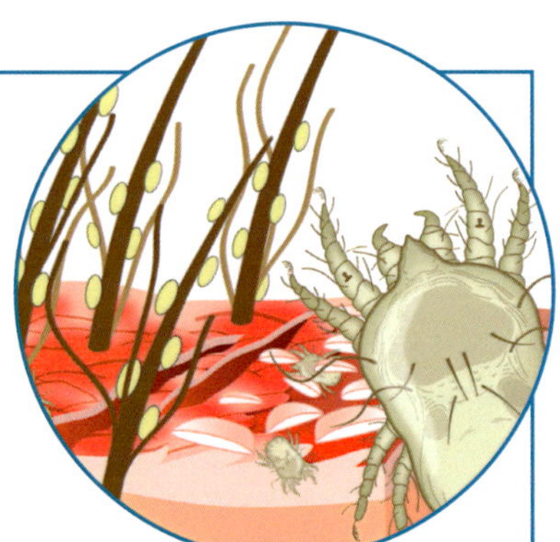

Cheyletiella

LICE

- Cat lice are *Felicola subrostrata* and cannot affect people.
- They are very uncommon.
- They mainly affect kittens living in poor conditions.

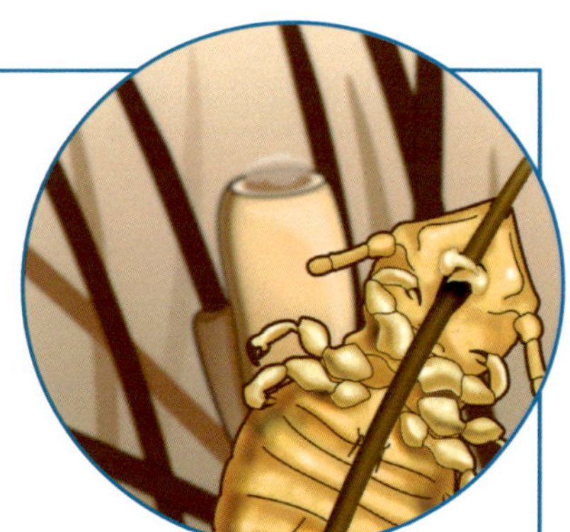

*The mites *Notoedres Cati* and *Otodectes cynotis* are seen in sheets 49 and 50 respectively.

DENTISTRY

53 Lesions of the mandible

Traumatic separation of the mandibular symphysis: repair by means of cerclage wire

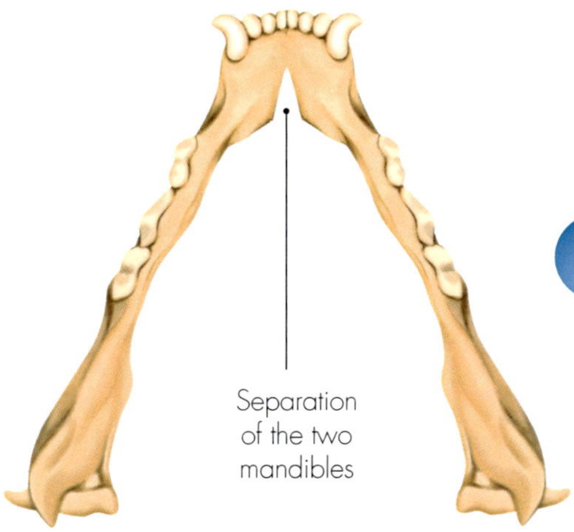

Cerclage wire

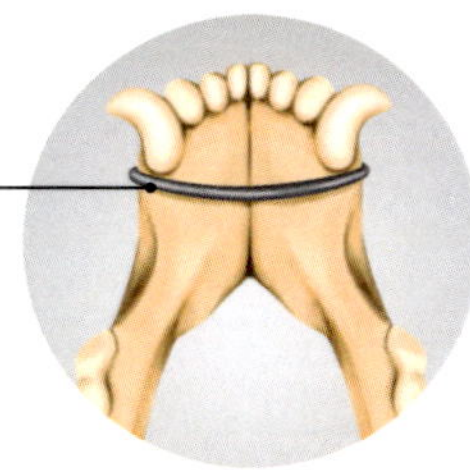

It may also be repaired by applying a splint from canine to canine with dentistry material.

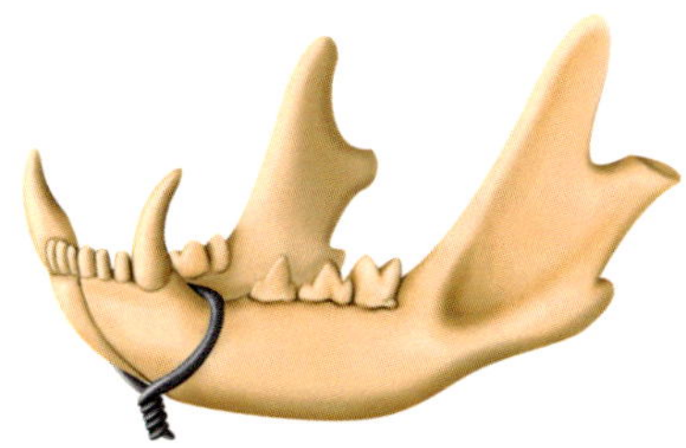

Temporomandibular joint luxation

Temporomandibular luxation is due to trauma (falls, road traffic accidents) and is almost always unilateral, although it may on occasions be bilateral. Luxation may be in a rostral dorsal or caudal ventral direction, the latter having a poorer prognosis as it is associated with fractures in the joint area.

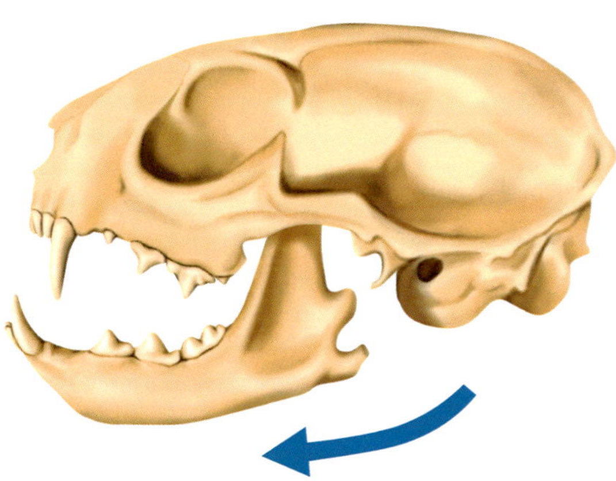

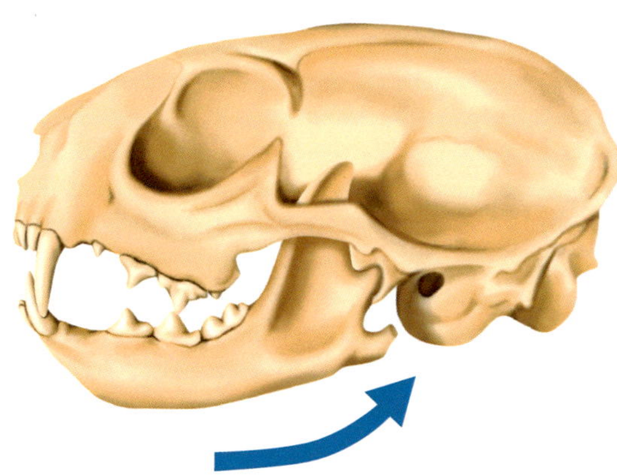

Medical treatment

Reduction of luxation and immobilisation of the area.

Surgical treatment

In cases in which the joint is fractured, due to the risk of ankylosis.

Clinical signs

- Dropped mandible and malocclusion.
- Inability to close the mouth.
- Hypersalivation.

DENTISTRY

54 Teeth in cats

Deciduous and permanent teeth

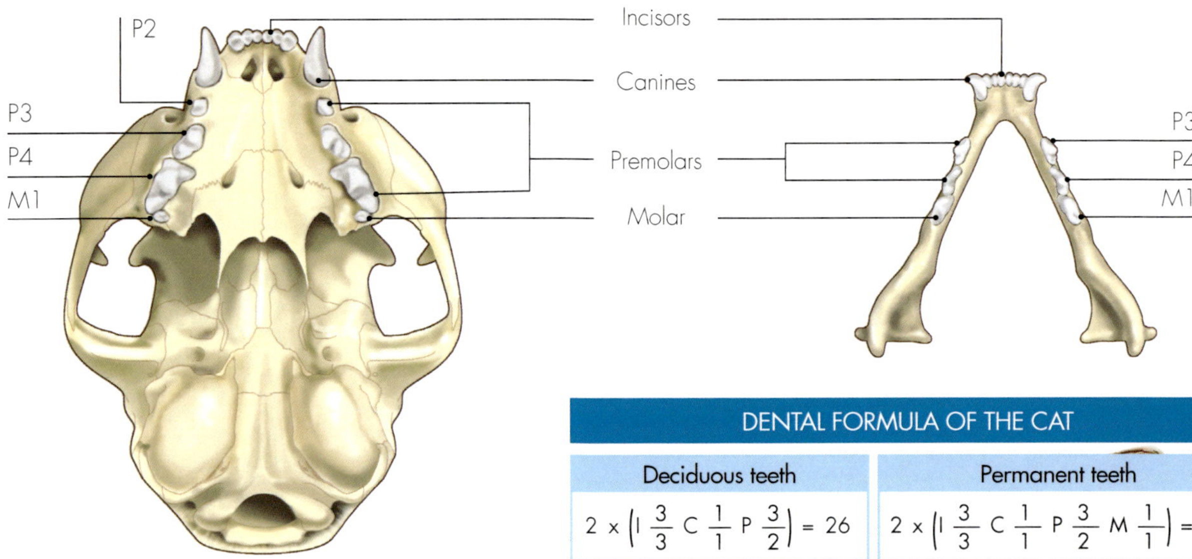

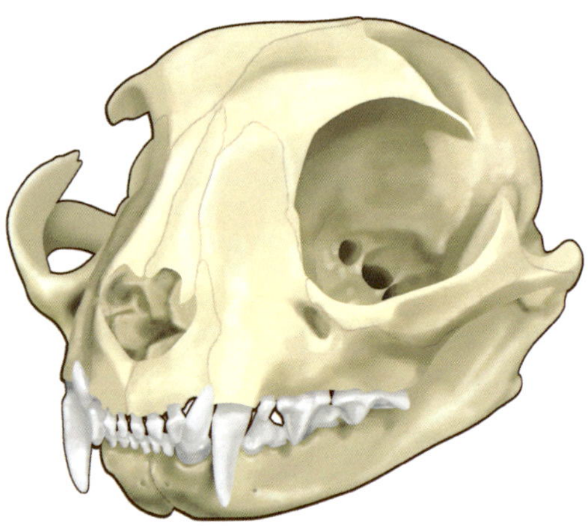

DENTAL FORMULA OF THE CAT	
Deciduous teeth	Permanent teeth
$2 \times \left(I \frac{3}{3}\ C \frac{1}{1}\ P \frac{3}{2} \right) = 26$	$2 \times \left(I \frac{3}{3}\ C \frac{1}{1}\ P \frac{3}{2}\ M \frac{1}{1} \right) = 30$

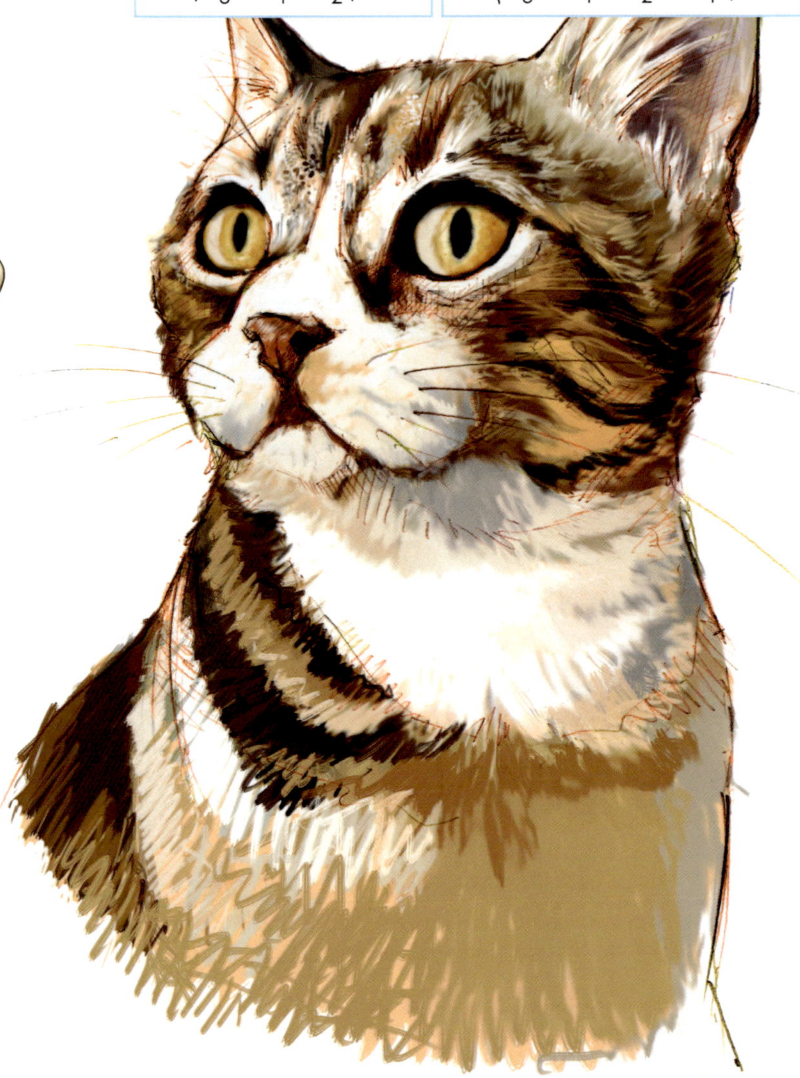

ERUPTION OF DECIDUOUS TEETH

- Incisors: 2–3 weeks.
- Canines: 3–4 weeks.
- Premolars: 3–6 weeks.
- Molars: absent.

ERUPTION OF PERMANENT TEETH

- Incisors: 3–4 months.
- Canines: 4–5 months.
- Premolars: 4–6 months.
- Molars: 4–5 months.
- Complete dentition at 6 months.

DENTISTRY

55 Periodontal disease

Periodontal disease is a condition caused by bacteria. It consists of two phases:

1. Gingivitis: initial phase caused by the accumulation of bacterial plaque (bacteria in biofilm) on the teeth over hours or days. Subsequently, the biofilm mineralises to form calculus (tartar). These bacteria provoke an inflammatory response leading to inflammation of the gums. **Treatment during this phase is curative.**
2. Periodontitis: due to chronic inflammation and the increased deposition of bacteria, the tissues that support the tooth are irreversibly damaged, and ultimately the tooth is lost. **Treatment does not repair the damaged tissues, but can prevent loss of the tooth.**

Stages

PHASE 1. Gingivitis.

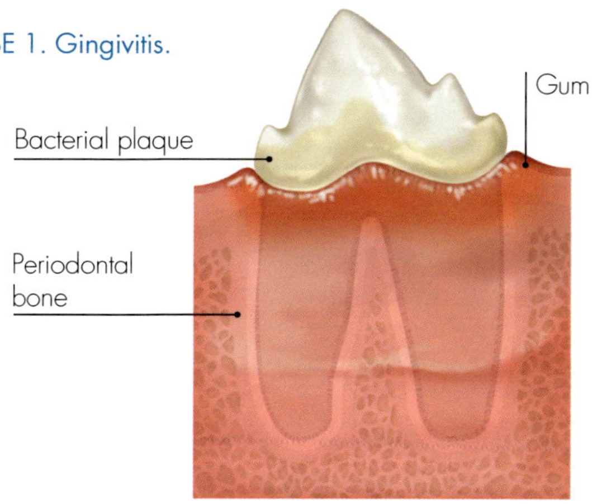

PHASE 2. Loss of 25 % of alveolar bone.

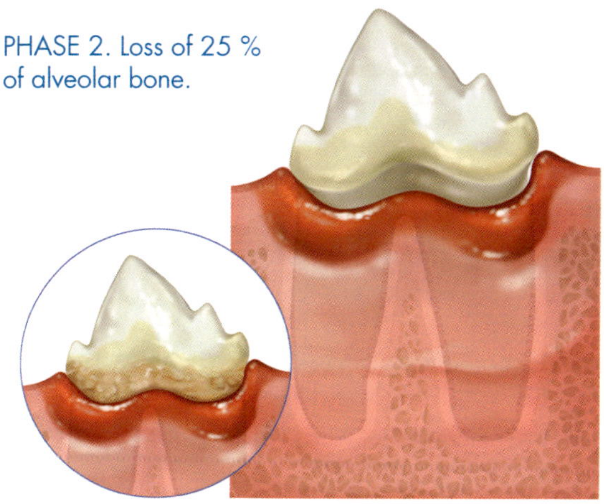

PHASE 3. Loss of 25–50 % of alveolar bone.

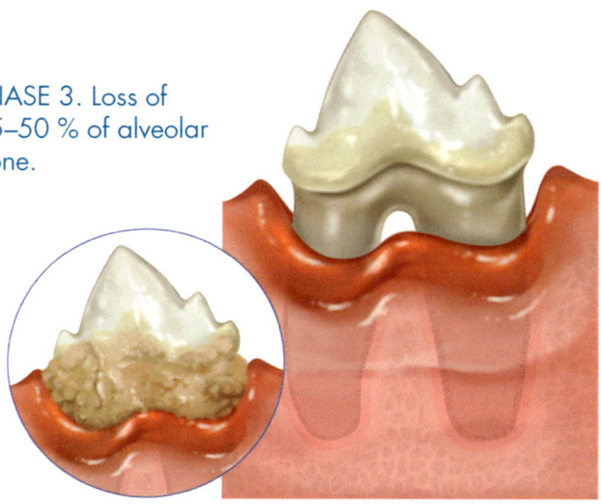

PHASE 4. Loss of >50 % of alveolar bone.

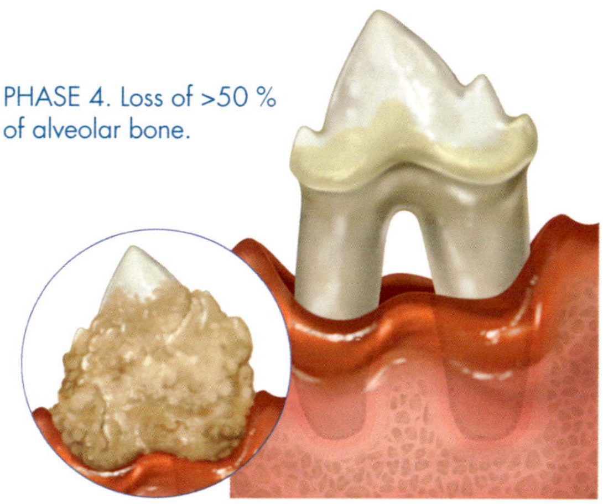

Treatment

Gingivitis:

- Dental cleaning and polishing in the clinic to remove calculus (tartar).
- Control of dental plaque at home by brushing and using toothpaste.

Periodontitis:

- Frequent dental cleaning and polishing.
- Dental radiographs to assess severity.
- Gingivectomy.
- Extraction of severely damaged teeth.

DENTISTRY

56 Tooth resorption in cats

False caries

It is one of the oral diseases with greater prevalence in cats all around the world. Its cause is still unknown, but it leads to the destruction of the dental tissue in the neck, root and crown of the tooth.

The lesions may be covered by dental plaque or by the inflamed gum, and may therefore go unnoticed. Owners usually do not notice them.

Dental radiographs are essential to determine the exact degree of the lesions.

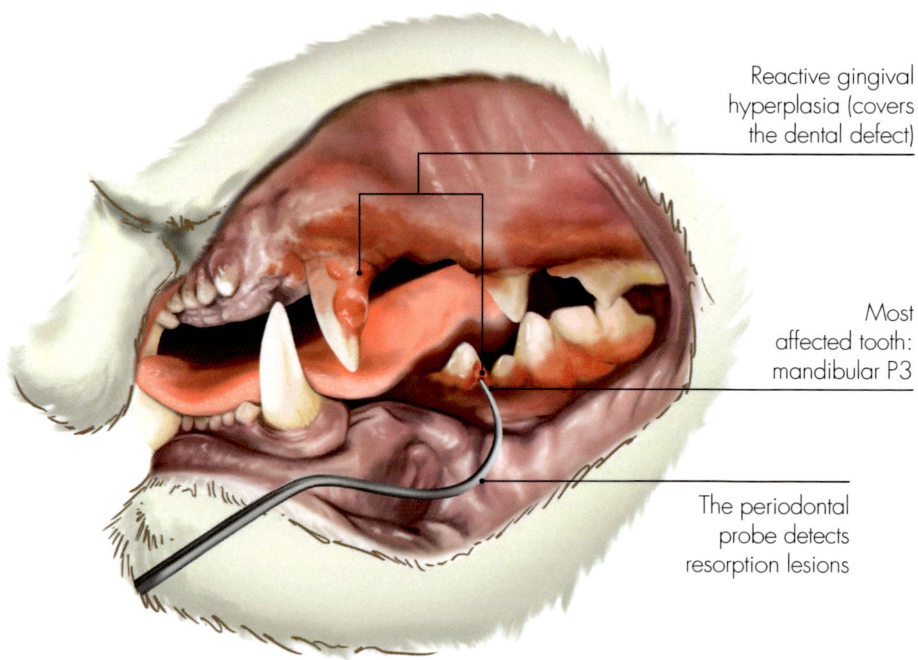

Tooth resorption causes pain during mastication. A common reason for the fact that many cats refuse to eat pills is the pain associated with this condition.

The American College of Veterinary Dentistry classifies dental resorption into five phases based on severity and location (class 1: no lesion)

CLASS 2

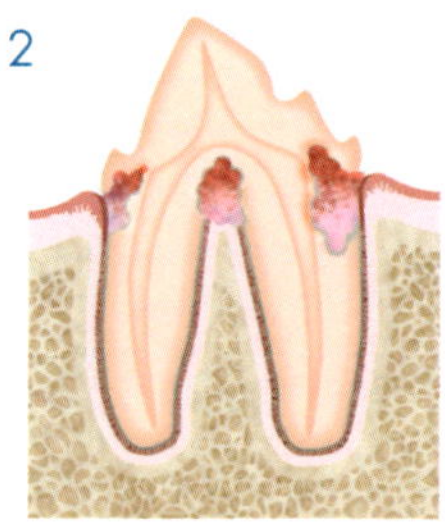

CLASS 3

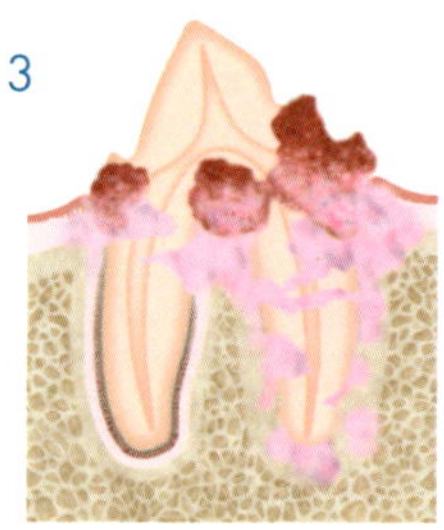

CLASS 4

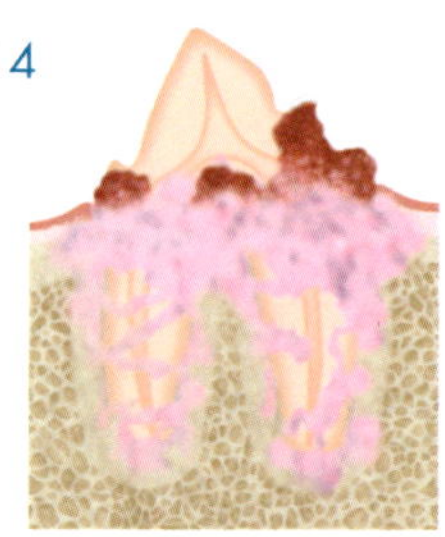

CLASS 5

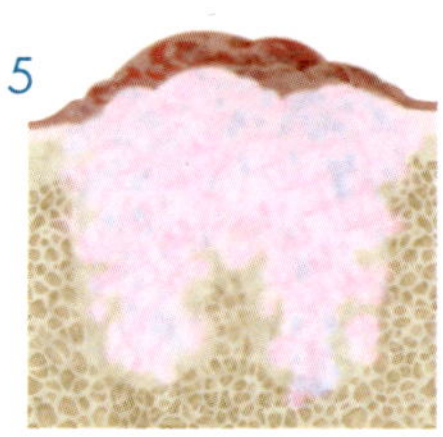

Medical treatment

There is no curative or preventive treatment.

Surgical treatment

Extraction is the technique of choice as it eliminates the pain caused by the affected teeth.

Clinical signs

- Changes in the behaviour and in dietary habits (affected cats prefer to eat soft food or stop eating).
- They may drool or show pain (they touch their mouth with their paws).

DENTISTRY

57 Feline chronic gingivostomatitis

Very painful ulcerative process, which affects all the tissues that are in contact with the saliva and bacterial plaque: gums, mucosae, palatoglossal arch and soft palate.

Diagnosis

- PCR for calicivirus of a sample of oral mucosa.
- Dental radiograph: tooth resorption or periodontal disease.
- Biopsies: only if there is unilateral involvement or proliferation (atypical cases).
- Bacterial culture of the palatoglossal arch in severe cases.

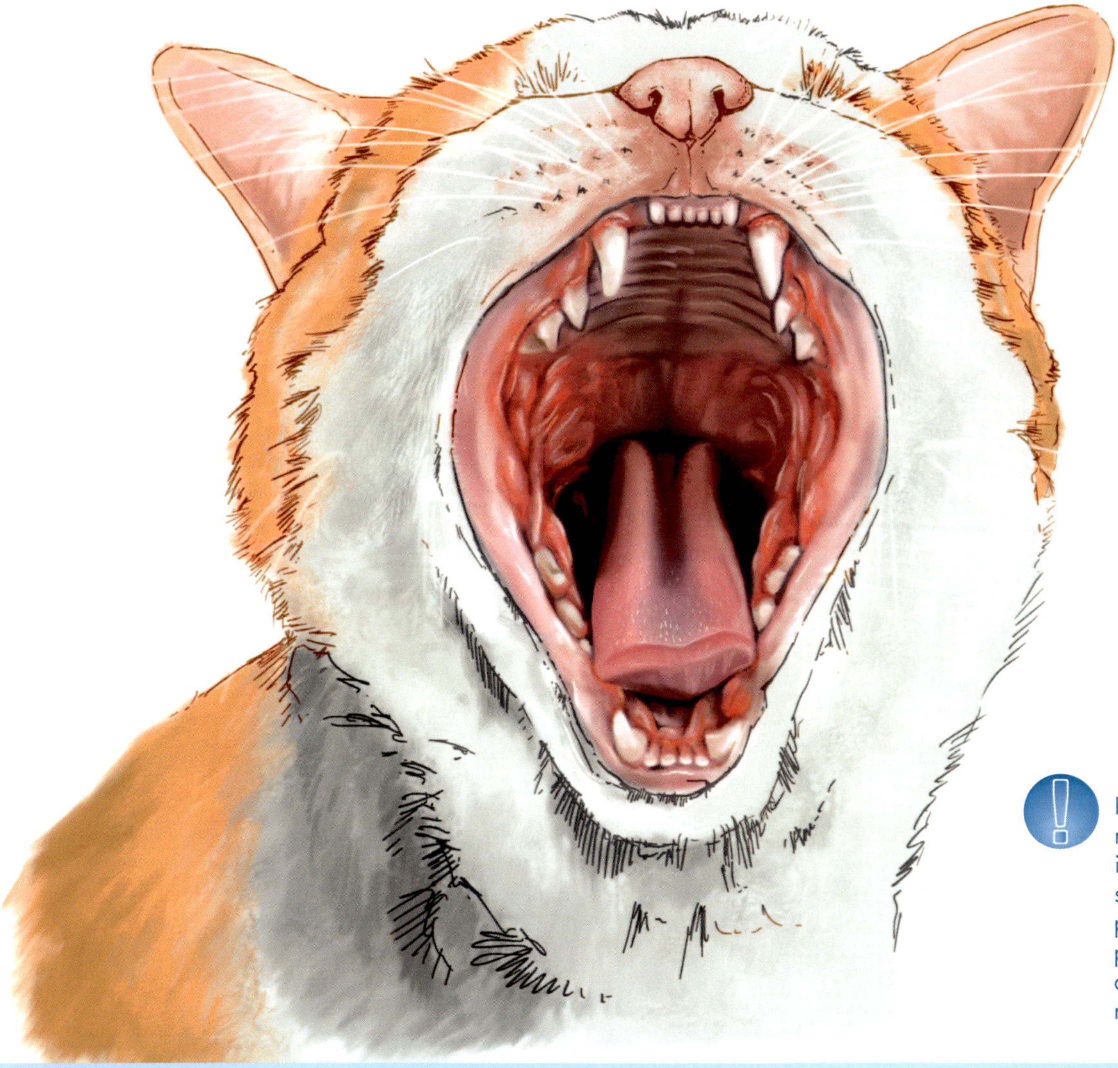

It is due to an exaggerated response of the local immune system to one or several of these conditions: presence of bacterial plaque, periodontal disease, calicivirus, tooth resorption.

Medical/surgical treatment

Varies in function of the cause and severity of the case:

- Pain control: NSAID and opiates.
- Periodontal disease: dental cleaning, extraction of the affected teeth and antibiotic therapy.
- Tooth resorption: extraction of the affected teeth.
- Calicivirus: immune modulators.

If there is no response to the treatment, or the clinical picture is initially very severe: extraction of all the teeth (except the canines, if possible), together with analgesics, antimicrobials and immune modulators.

In cases in which extraction does not result in improvement, stem cell therapy can provide good results.

DIGESTIVE SYSTEM

58 Feline gastrointestinal inflammatory disease

Group of gastrointestinal disorders characterised by inflammation of the digestive mucosa. Multifactorial origin: genetic and immune alterations and alterations of the digestive bacterial flora.

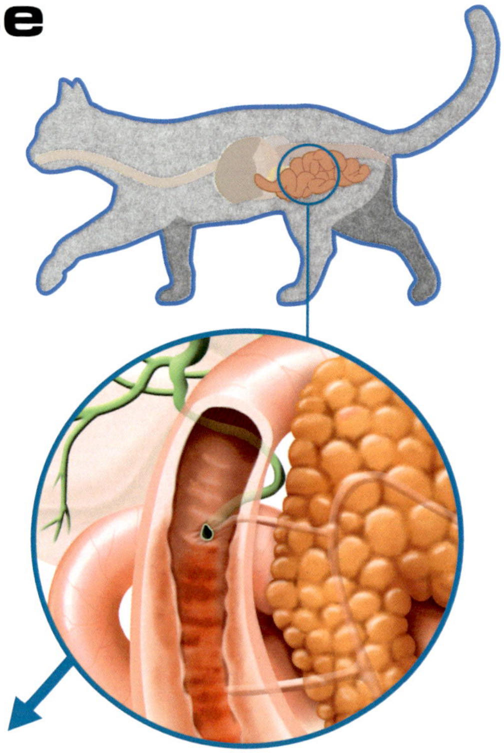

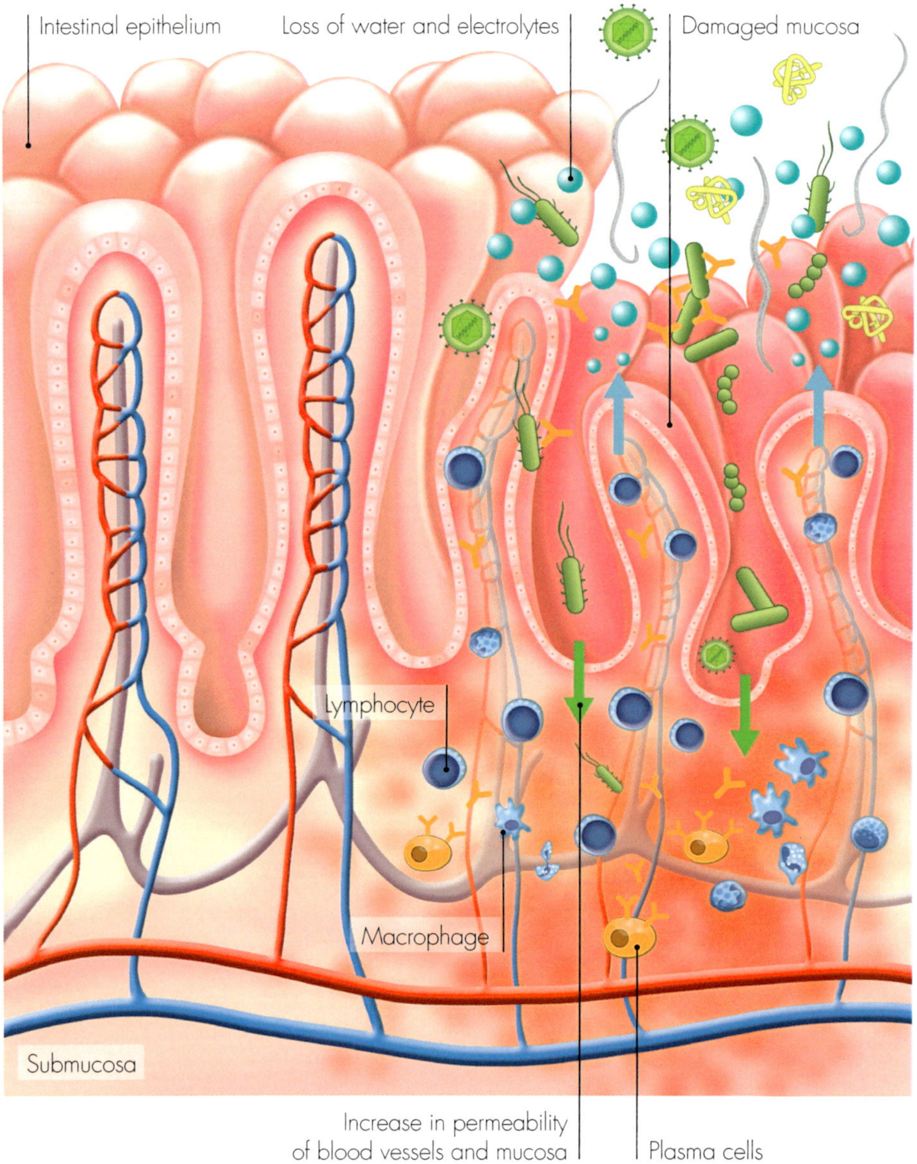

Clinical signs

- Chronic gastrointestinal signs (more than 3 weeks) with variable severity (periods of improvement and periods of relapse): vomiting, diarrhoea, anorexia, loss of weight, disorders of the appetite.
- No response to dietary modifications or symptomatic treatments.

It is the disease most frequently diagnosed in cats with vomiting and/or chronic diarrhoea.

Diagnosis

- Rule out other causes of intestinal inflammation: parasites, endocrinopathies, adverse reaction to food, etc.
- Biopsy of the stomach, duodenum, jejunum, and ileum by endoscopy or surgery (laparoscopy or laparotomy).

Medical treatment

- Corticosteroids.
- Metronidazole.
- Mesenchymal stem cell therapy.

Dietary treatment

Hypoallergenic diet (novel or hydrolysate).

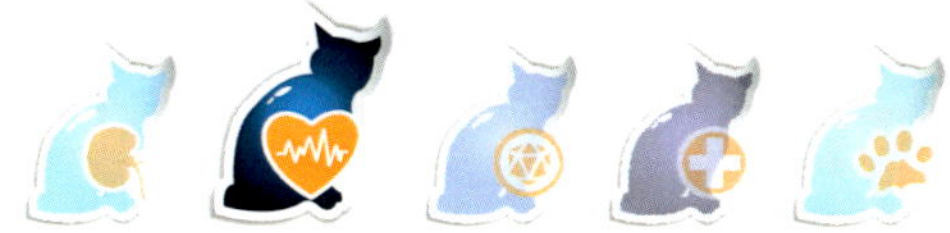

DIGESTIVE SYSTEM

59 Low-grade lymphoma

Low-grade lymphoma (LGL) is a T-cell tumour that originates in the base of the intestinal villi and mainly affects cats aged >8 years. Currently, LGL accounts for 10–13 % of all feline lymphomas.

Clinical signs

- Signs are the same as those observed for IBD, including vomiting and/or chronic diarrhoea.
- However, in some cats progressive weight loss together with a good appetite is the main sign.

Diagnosis

- Like inflammatory bowel disease (IBD), diagnosis requires ruling out other diseases that cause chronic digestive signs.
- Biopsy:
  - Digestive endoscopy with biopsy of the duodenum, jejunum, and ileum.
  - Laparoscopy or laparotomy, if liver or pancreas biopsy are also required.

It is common for LGL to affect one intestinal tract, while the others are affected by IBD. Hence, all intestinal segments must be biopsied: duodenum, jejunum, and ileum.

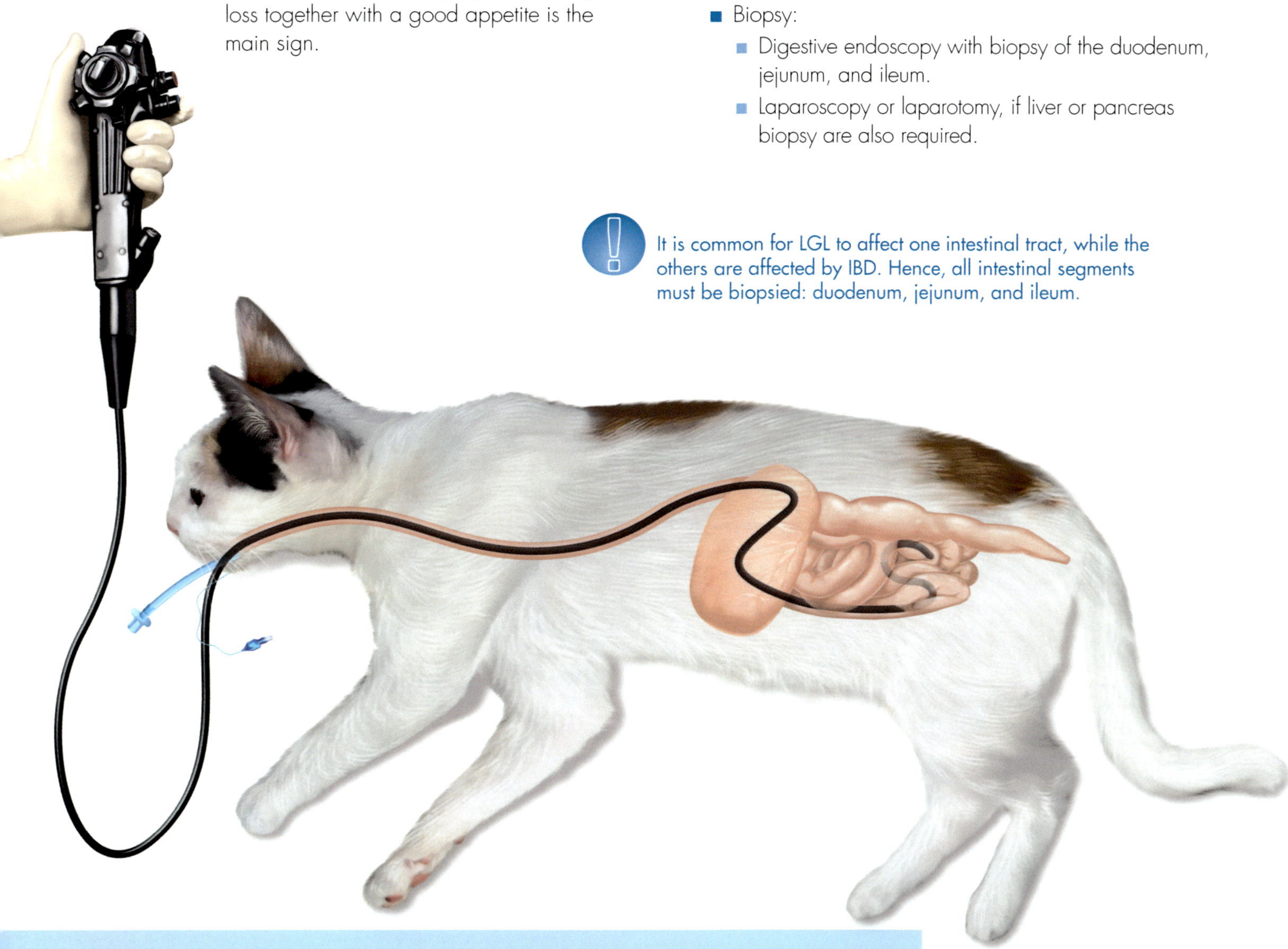

Treatment

With proper treatment, consisting of the administration of prednisolone and chlorambucil, survival time is very long (>2 years) and the patient can maintain good quality of life.

DIGESTIVE SYSTEM

60 Hepatic lipidosis

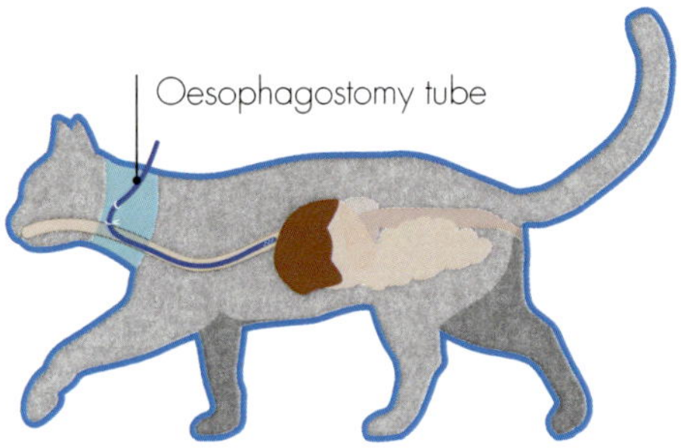

It is the accumulation of lipids in the cytoplasm of hepatocytes, which leads to improper functioning of the liver. It is the most frequent hepatic disease in cats.

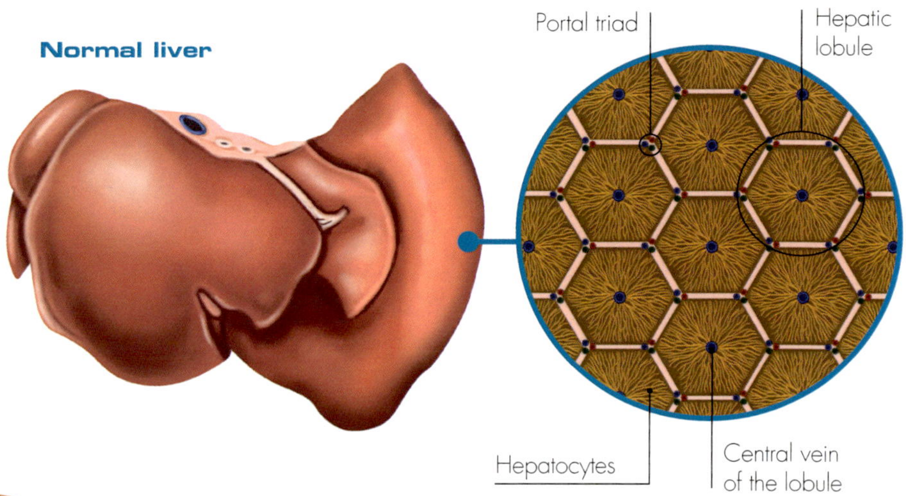

Most cats affected by hepatic lipidosis are obese before becoming sick.

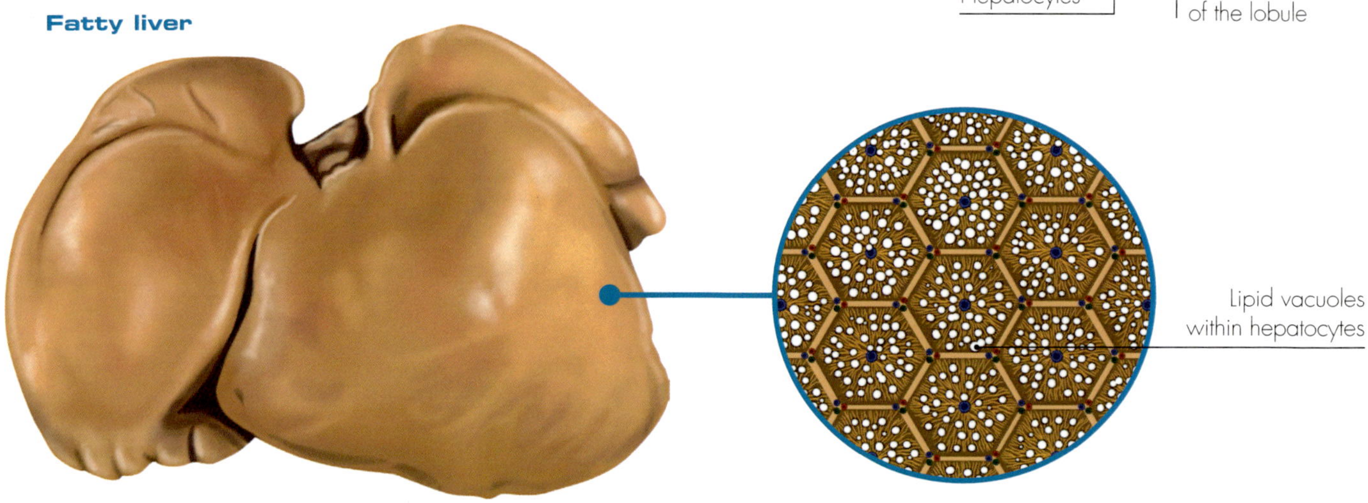

Causes

- It occurs during periods of prolonged hyporexia, with accumulated weight loss of approximately 30 %.
- Lipidosis occurs secondary to another disease that causes hyporexia. The most frequent causes are cholangitis, inflammatory bowel disease, and pancreatitis.

Clinical signs

- Jaundice (yellowish pigmentation of the sclerae, mucosae and soft palate), anorexia and depression with intermittent vomiting.
- Other clinical signs such as ascites (free abdominal fluid) and fever are less frequent.

Medical treatment

Although the disease may be fatal, more than 60 % of cats recover with intensive nutritional therapy by means of an oesophagostomy tube and medical treatment.

DIGESTIVE SYSTEM

61 Cholangitis

Cholangitis is an inflammation of the bile ducts. There are two forms of cholangitis: the neutrophilic form, which is caused by the passage of bacteria from the intestine to the biliary tract, and the lymphocytic form, due to an immune-mediated process.

Bacteria can also spread from the intestine to the pancreas and liver by haematogenous route.

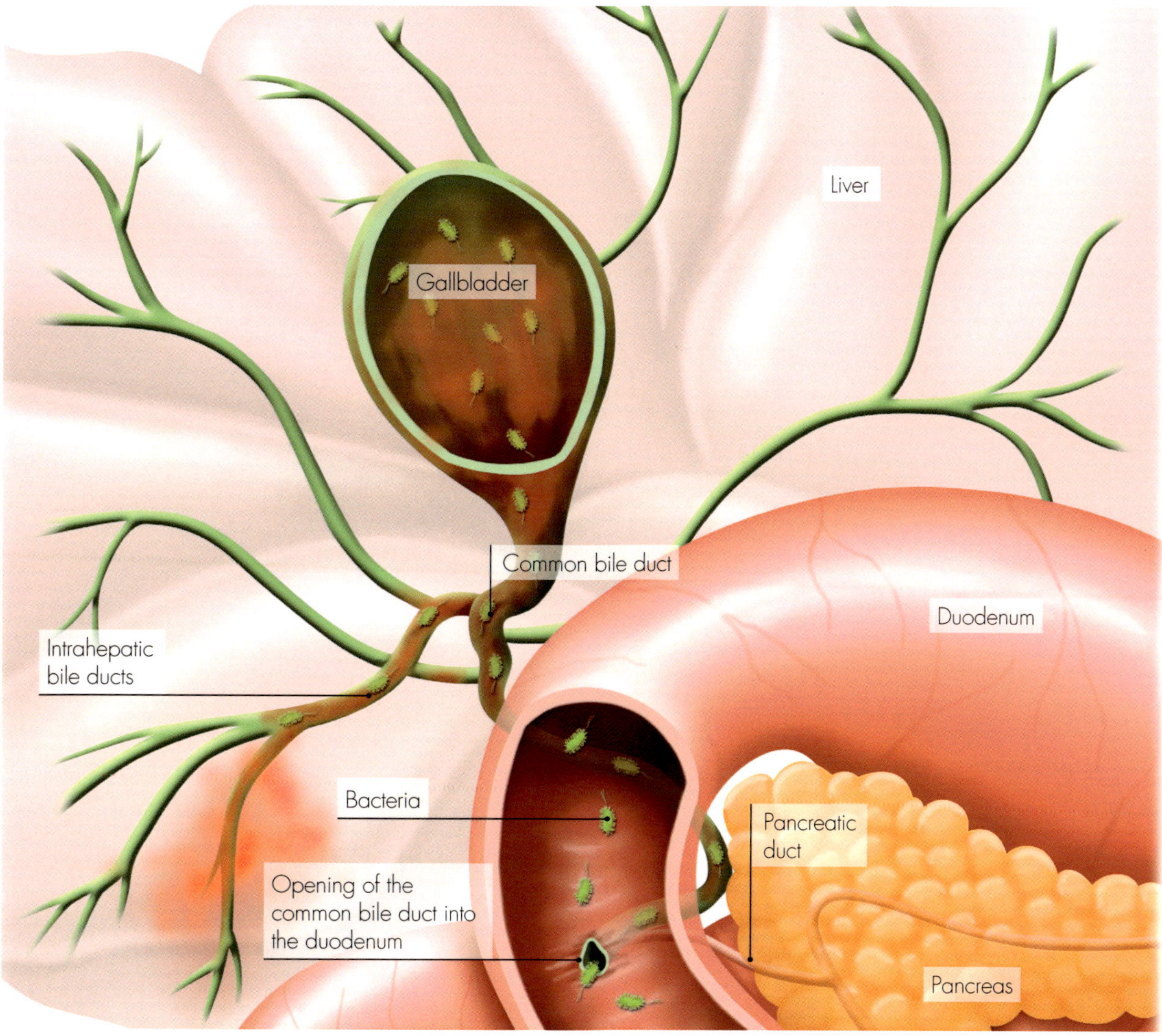

Clinical signs

- Anorexia and lack of energy.
- Loss of weight.
- Fever in the case of neutrophilic cholangitis.
- Jaundice.
- Hepatomegaly.
- Free abdominal fluid, especially in cases of lymphocytic cholangitis.

Diagnosis

It requires multiple tests to differentiate both conditions:

- Blood analysis (liver function).
- Abdominal ultrasound scan.
- Bile culture.
- Collection of biopsies (ultrasound-guided or by means of laparoscopy or laparotomy).

DIGESTIVE SYSTEM

62 Pancreatitis and triaditis

Triaditis is the concurrence of pancreatitis, intestinal inflammatory process and cholangitis. It occurs because, in cats, the pancreatic duct joins the common bile duct before opening into the duodenum.

This condition is caused by the reflux of bacteria from the duodenum through the common bile duct to the pancreas and liver. In some cases bacterial translocation is the cause.

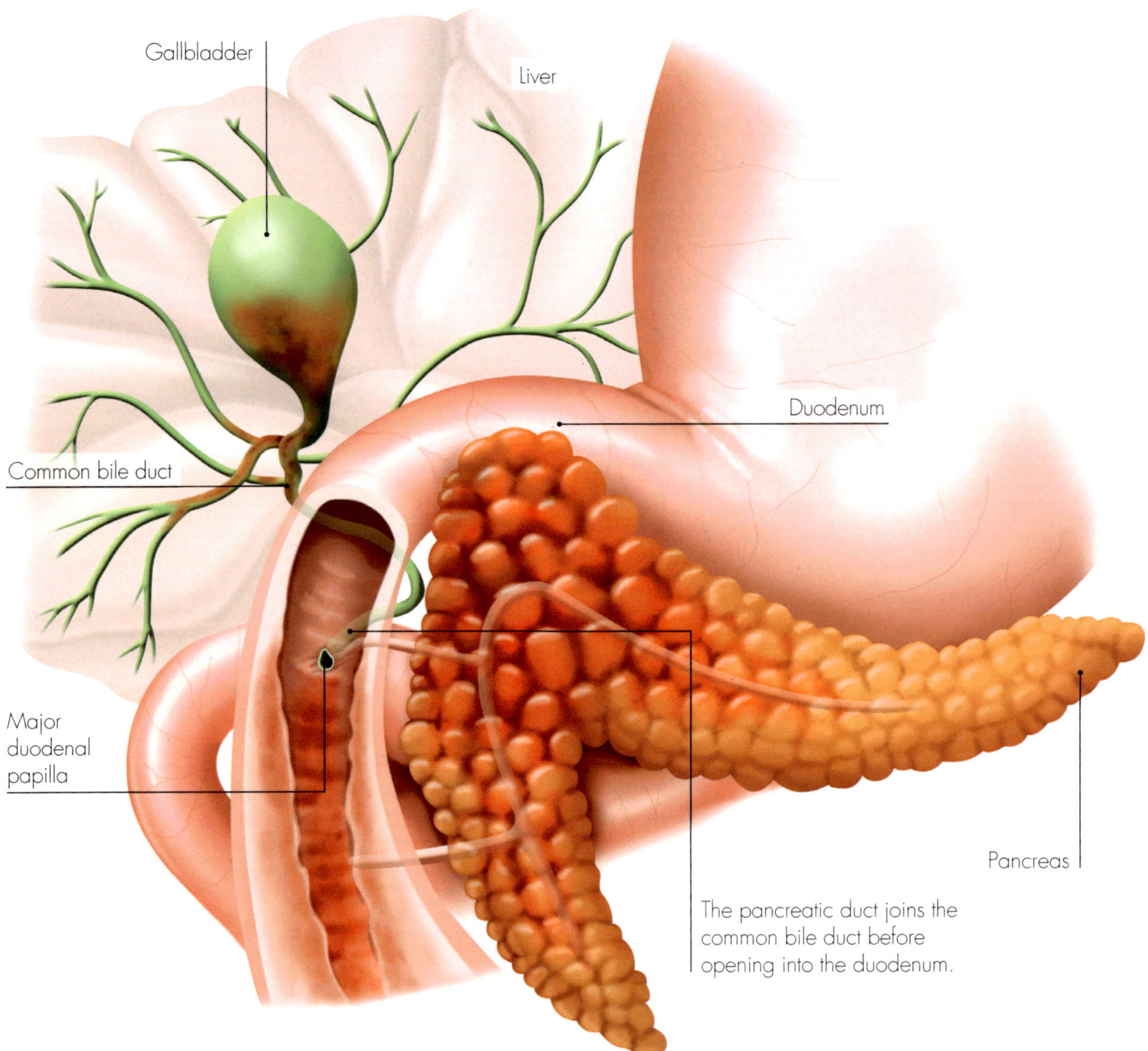

Causes of pancreatitis

- Drugs and toxic substances (organophosphates)
- Infectious agents: *Toxoplasma gondii,* hypervirulent calicivirus, FIP virus, panleukopaenia virus, herpesvirus.
- Trauma.
- Hypotension.
- Obstruction due to neoplasm.
- Duodenal reflux caused by intestinal inflammatory reflux.
- Biliary reflux caused by cholangitis.

Clinical signs

- Very variable.
- Depression, chronic vomiting and loss of weight are the most frequent signs.
- Other: diarrhoea, dehydration, jaundice, and in severe cases dyspnoea, abdominal pain and shock.

DIGESTIVE SYSTEM

63 Intestinal obstruction due to trichobezoars

Hairballs

Trichobezoars form throughout the gastrointestinal system of cats as a consequence of hair ingestion during daily grooming. However, it is not normal for cats to vomit hairballs. More than 75 % of short-haired cats and up to 50 % of long-haired cats never vomit.

The frequent elimination of trichobezoars used to be considered normal, while this is in fact wrong.

Sign of disease

The frequent elimination of trichobezoars, especially in short-haired cats, is a sign of:

- Inflammatory digestive problem: gastrointestinal inflammatory disease, adverse reaction to food, etc .
- Cutaneous problem: increased grooming (external parasites, hypersensitivity, etc.).

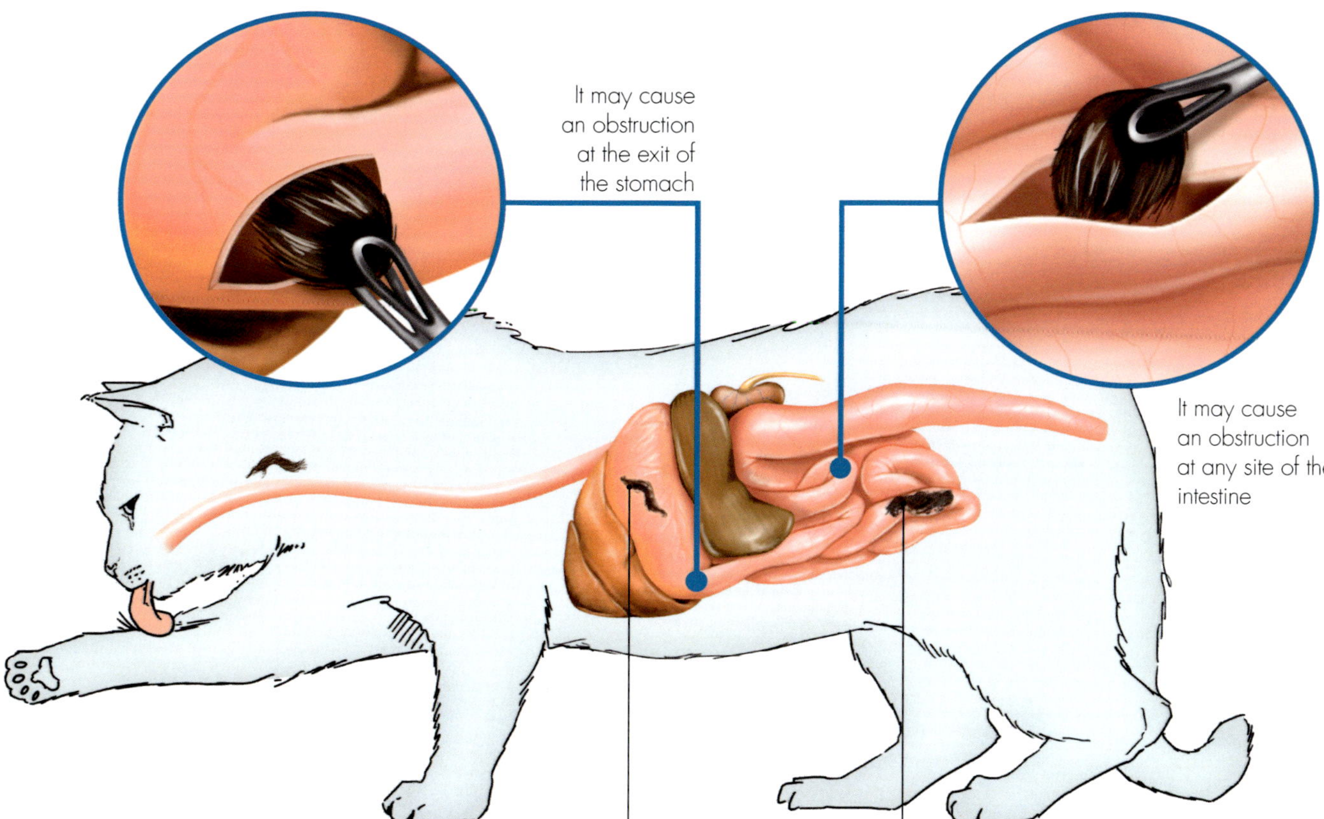

In the event that the frequency of vomiting increases, digestive disease should be suspected.

Surgical treatment

Severe obstruction: removal by means of surgery or endoscopy.

Recommendations:

- Diagnosis of digestive or dermatological diseases.
- Frequent brushing, especially in long-haired breeds and during the shedding season.
- Fibre-rich diets or specific diets to reduce the formation of trichobezoars.

DIGESTIVE SYSTEM

64 Megacolon

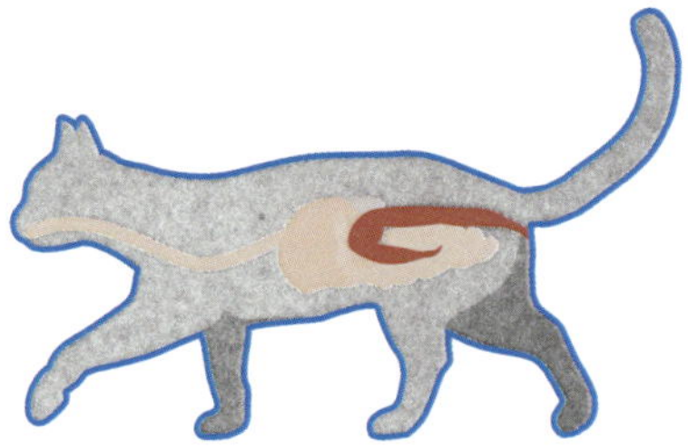

Megacolon is defined as a dilation of the large intestine. A functional anomaly of the colon causes faecal material to accumulate and prevents its elimination.

If the maximum diameter of the colon/the length of L5 >1.6 on the radiograph → diagnosis of megacolon.

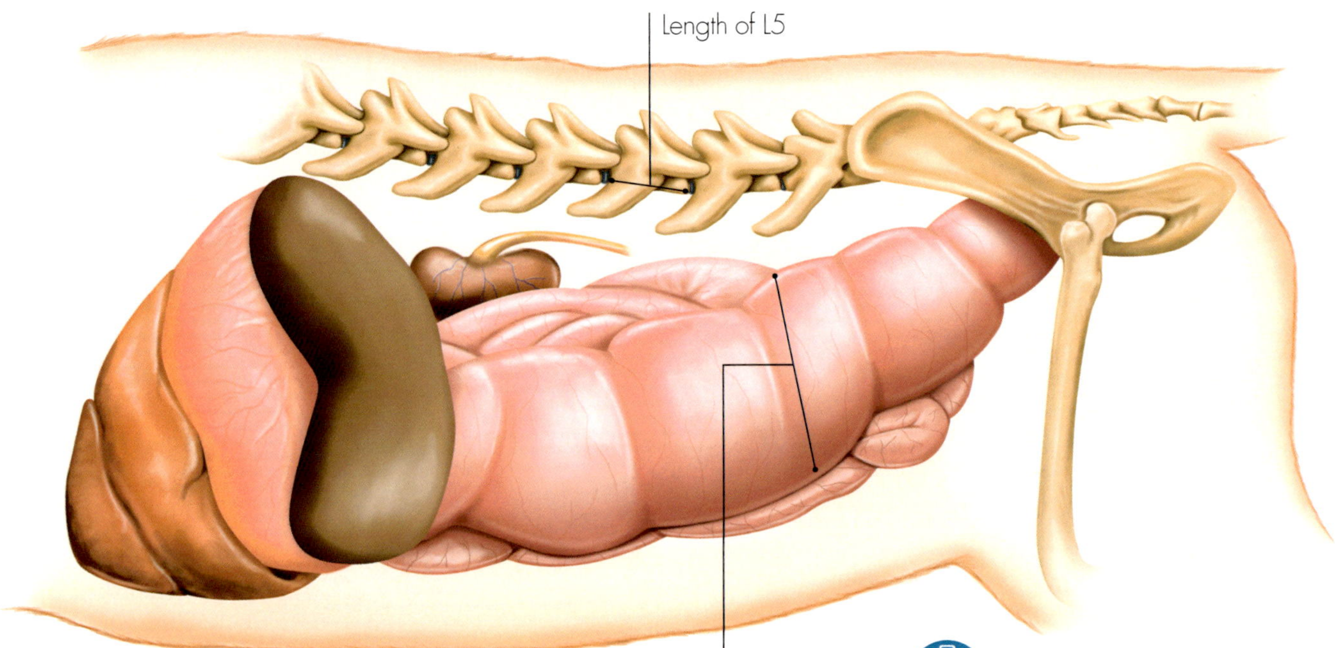

The diagnosis requires abdominal and hip radiographs as well as a neurological examination.

Classification

- **Congenital:** due to problems in the development of some of the segments caused by anatomical abnormalities or neurological development problems.
- **Secondary to an obstruction:** due to stenosis, masses, neoplasms, etc.
- **Idiopathic megacolon:** generally in cats from 8 years old. Dysfunction of the smooth muscle of the colon leading to severe chronic constipation and subsequently megacolon.

Clinical signs

- Chronic constipation.
- Tenesmus: painful and unproductive attempts to defecate (meows).
- Faeces out of the litter tray (aversion due to pain).
- Bloody fluid similar to diarrhoea (irritation of the mucosa).
- Vomiting in severe clinical pictures, due to irritation of the colon and absorption of toxins.
- Anorexia, lethargy and weakness.

Medical treatment

- Enemas in cases of severe constipation.
- Laxatives by oral route.
- Prokinetic drugs such as ranitidine.

Surgical treatment

- Applied if the drug therapy is not effective.
- Subtotal colectomy is the technique of choice, 85–95 % of the colon is removed.

Dietary treatment

Diets rich in insoluble fibres.

DIGESTIVE SYSTEM

65 Most common feline intestinal parasites

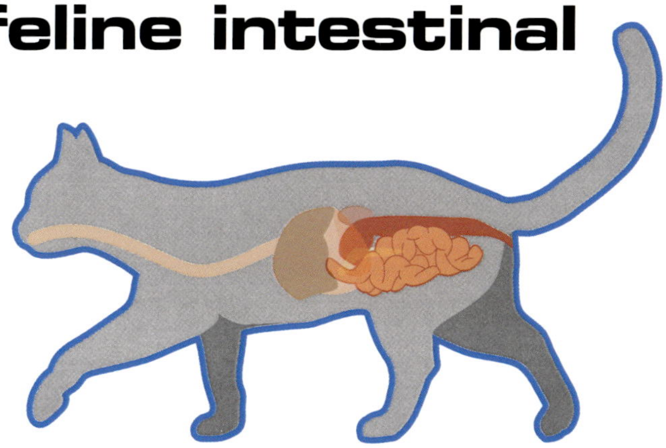

Disease transmissible to humans (zoonosis).

Protozoa

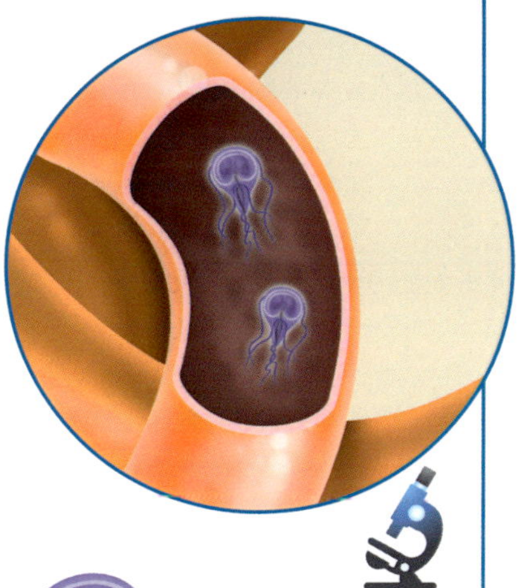

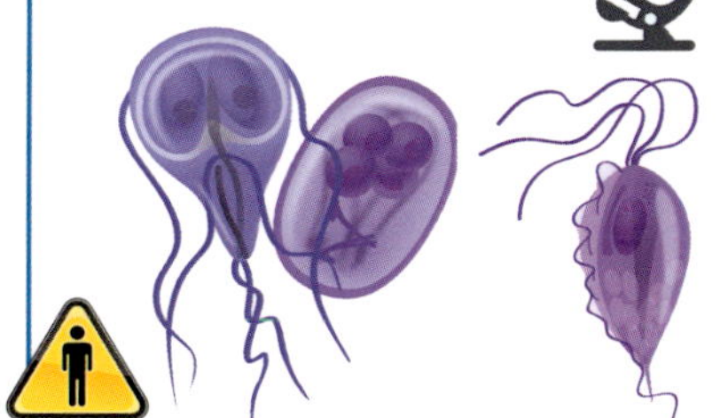

Giardia *Tritrichomonas*

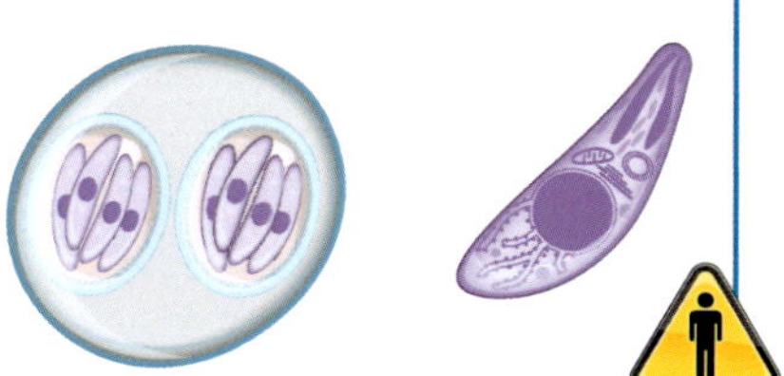

Isospora *Toxoplasma*

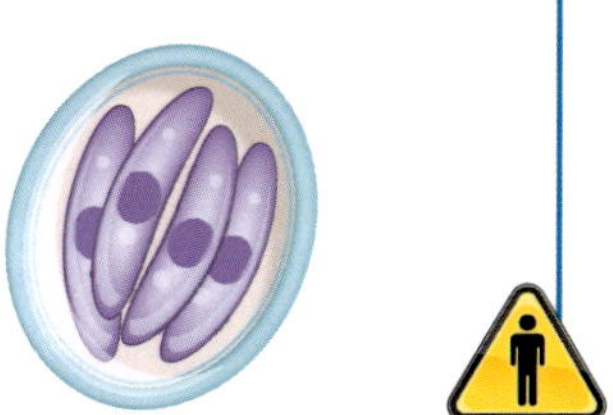

Cryptosporidium

Nematodes

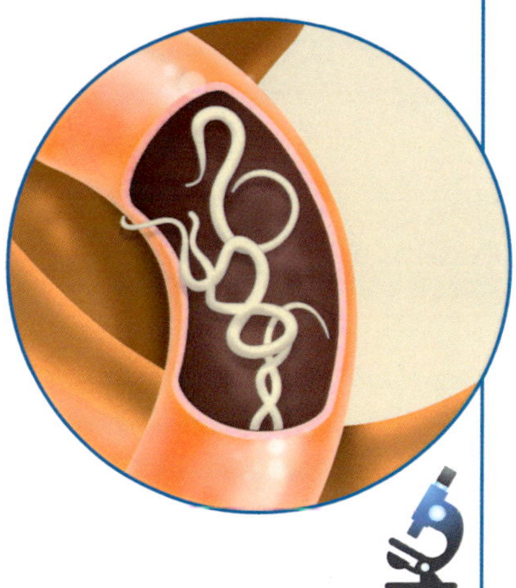

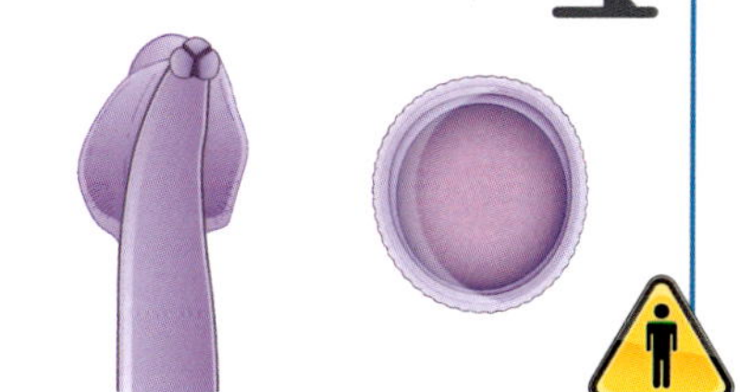

Toxocara cati

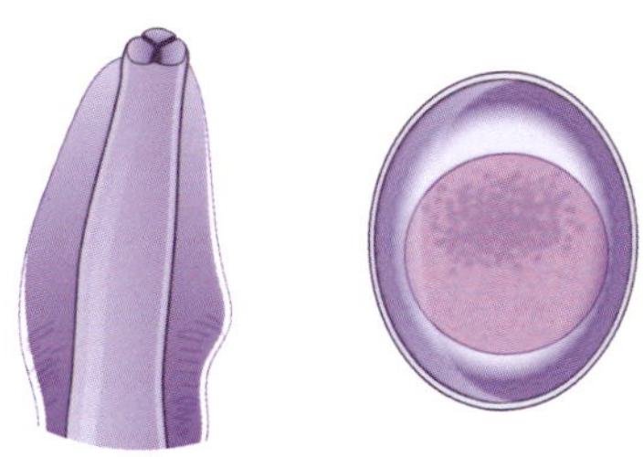

Toxascaris leonina

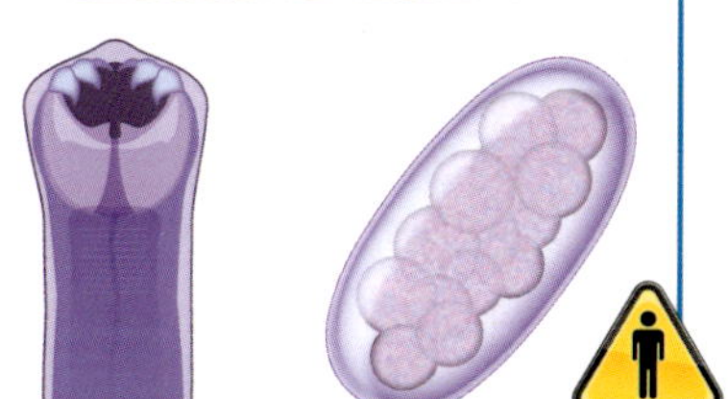

Ancylostoma tubaeforme

Cestodes

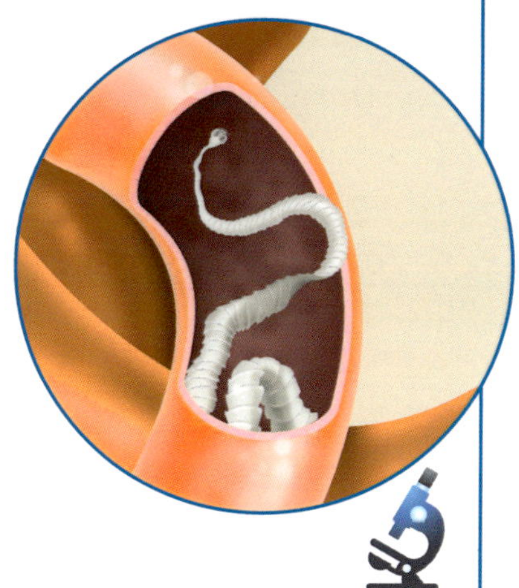

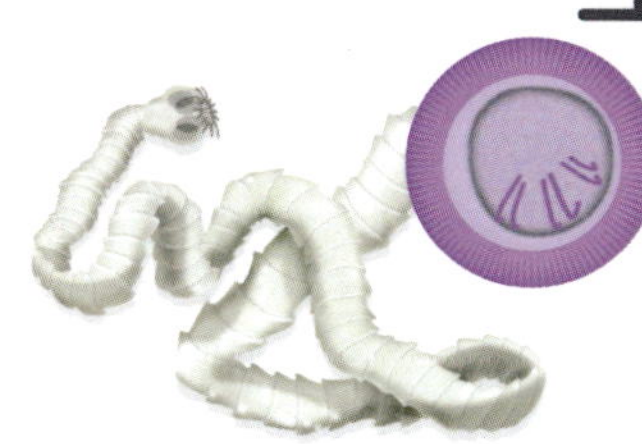

Taenia spp.

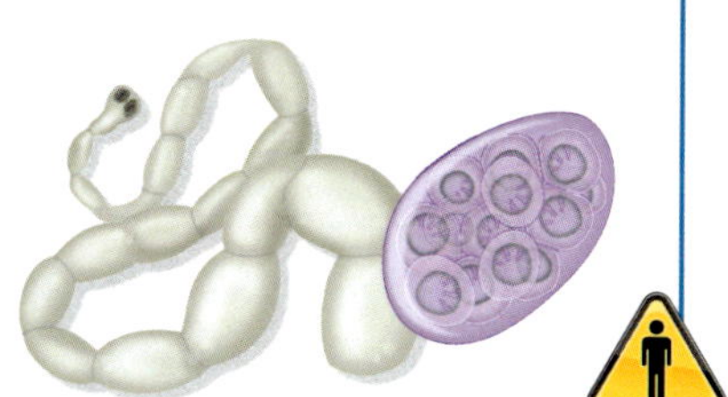

Dypilidium caninum

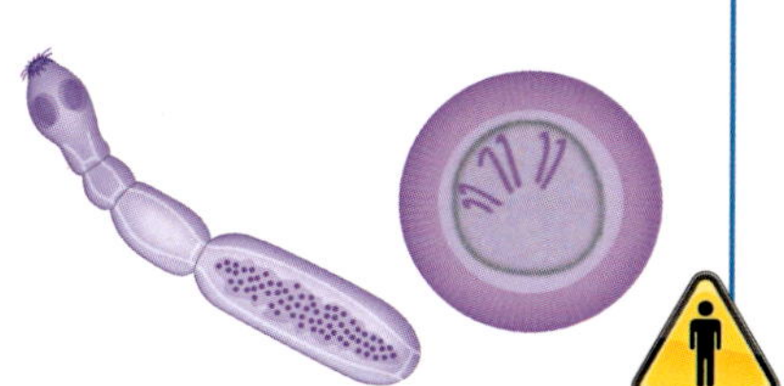

Echinococcus multilocularis

NERVOUS SYSTEM

66 Central, peripheral and autonomic nervous system

CENTRAL NERVOUS SYSTEM

1. Brain
2. Cerebellum
3. Spinal cord
4. Brainstem
5. 5th lumbar vertebra
6. 6th lumbar vertebra
7. Spinal cord
8. Cauda equina

PERIPHERAL NERVOUS SYSTEM

9. Cervical spinal nerves
10. Brachial plexus (C5, C6, C7, T1)
11. Radial n.
12. Musculocutaneous n.
13. Median n.
14. Ulnar n.
15. Thoracic spinal nerves
16. Lumbar spinal nerves
17. Lumbar plexus (L5, L6, L7, S1, S2)
18. Femoral n.
19. Saphenous n.
20. Obturator n.
21. Ischial n.

AUTONOMIC NERVOUS SYSTEM

22. Cranial cervical ganglion
23. Distal vagal ganglion
24. Vagosympathetic trunk
25. Caudal cervical ganglion
26. Cervicothoracic ganglion
27. Vagus n.
28. Vagus n., dorsal branch
29. Vagus n., ventral branch
30. Ganglia of the sympathetic trunk
31. Celiac-mesenteric ganglion
32. Caudal mesenteric ganglion
33. Hypogastric n.

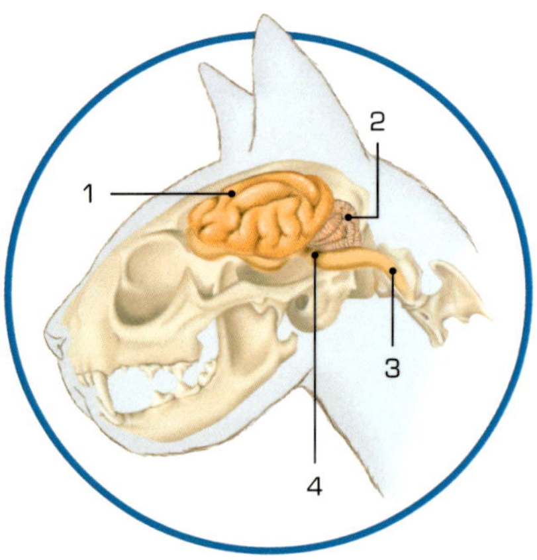

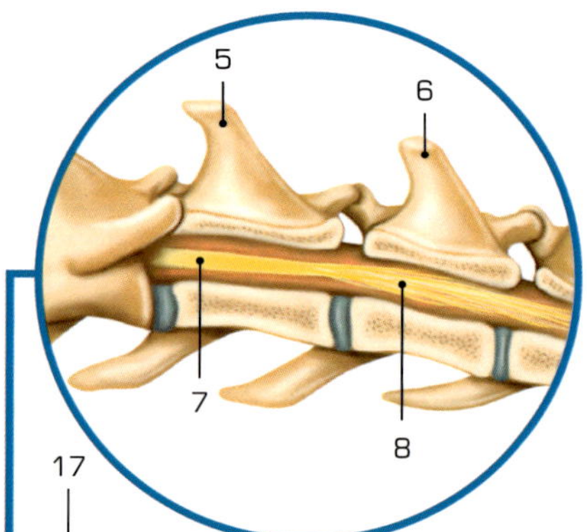

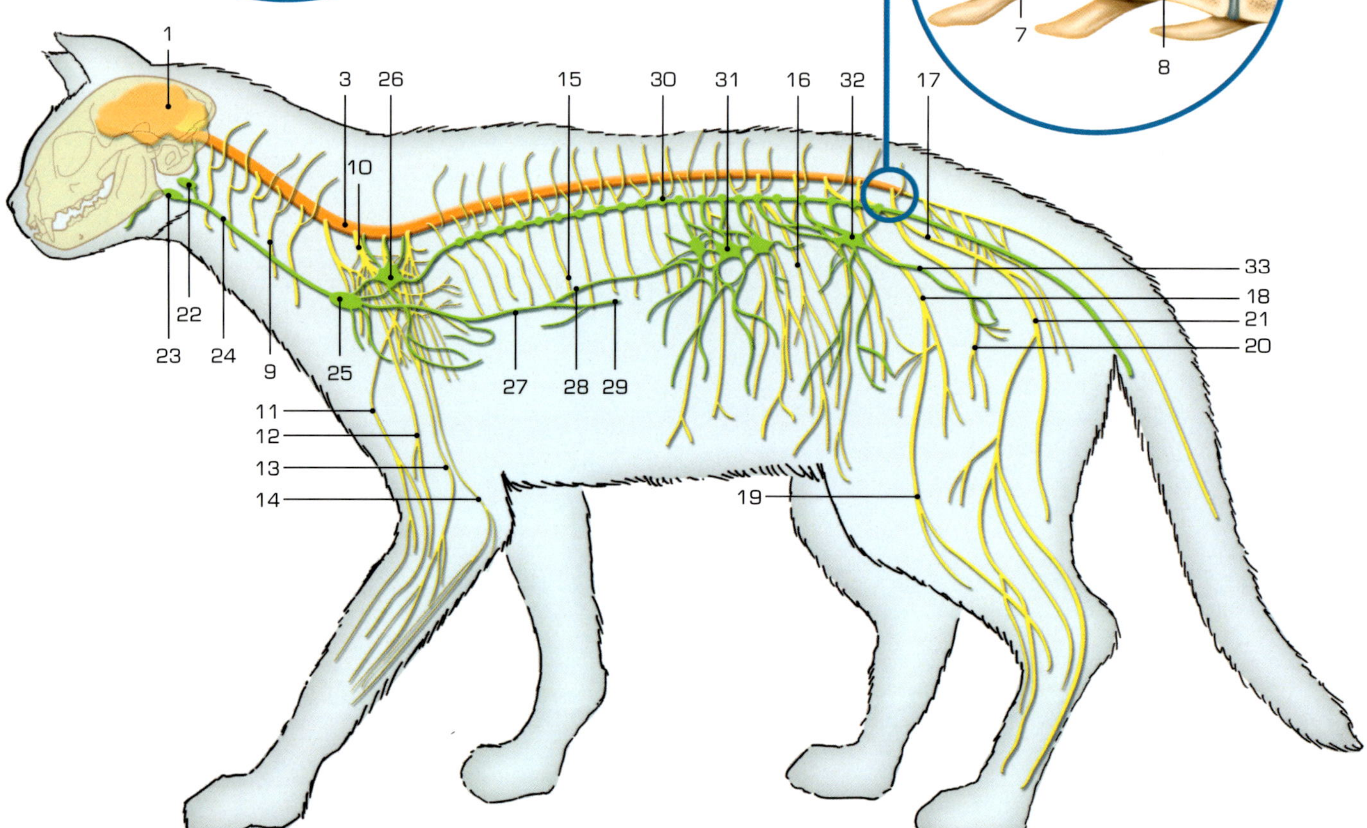

EYES

67 Structures of the eye

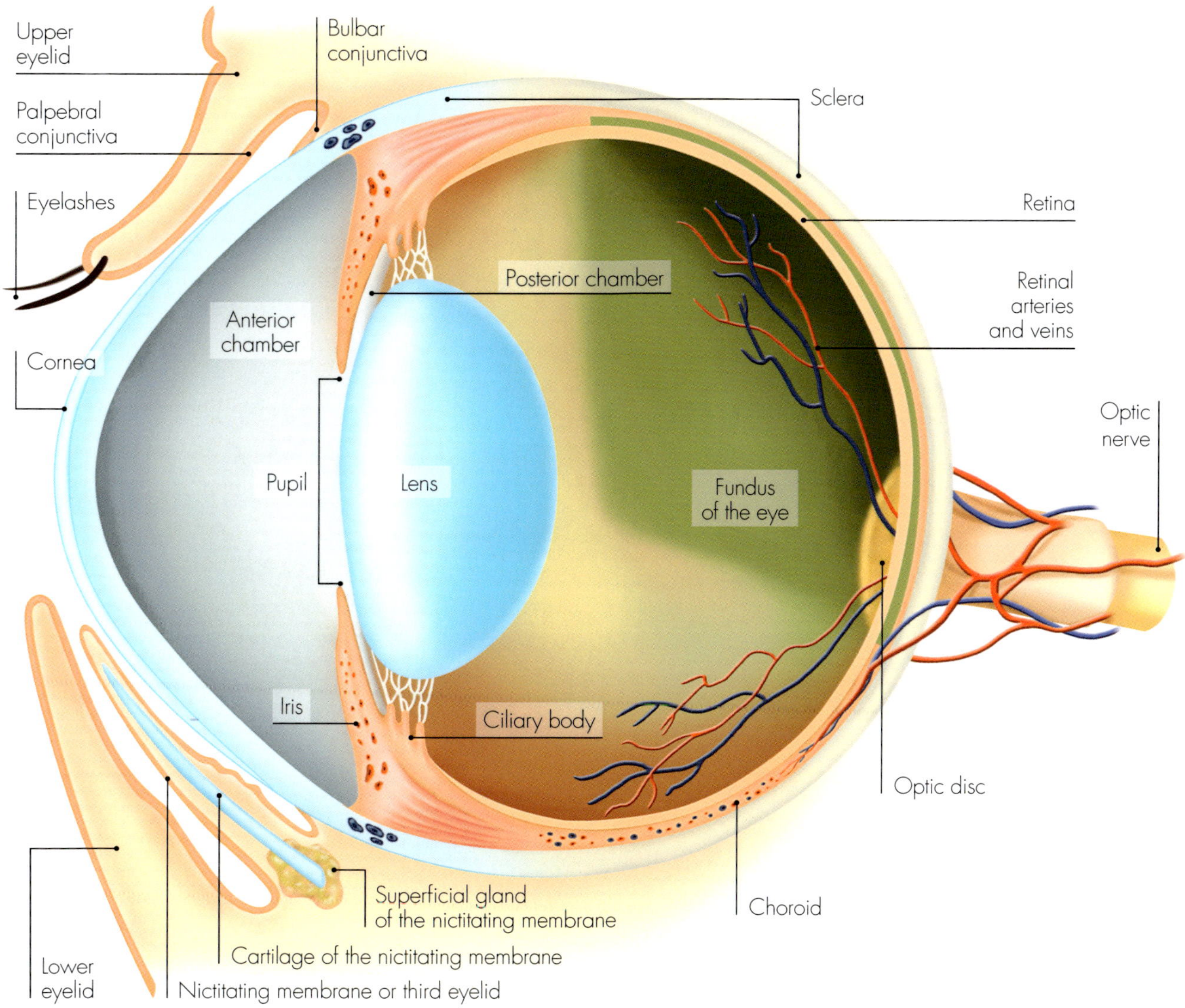

Mechanism of pupillary reflex

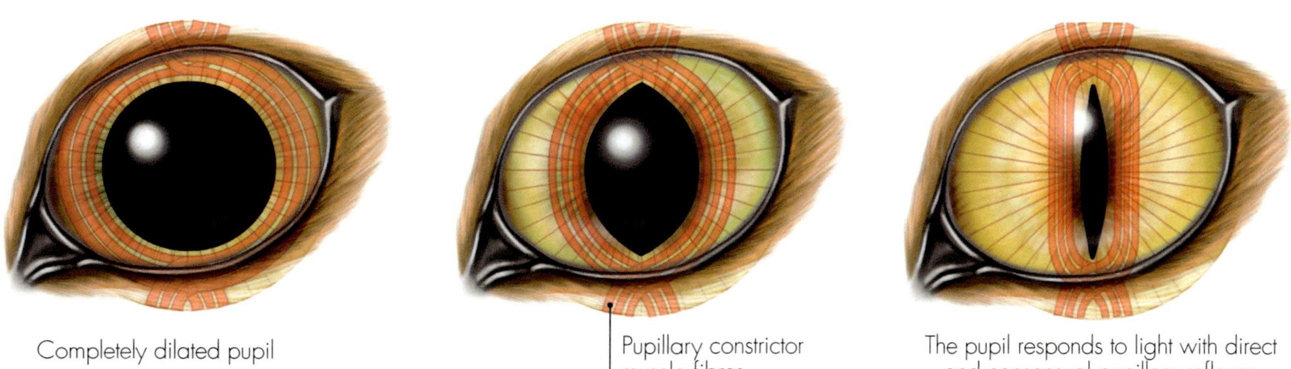

EYES

68 Corneal ulcer and keratitis

Surgical treatment of severe ulcers

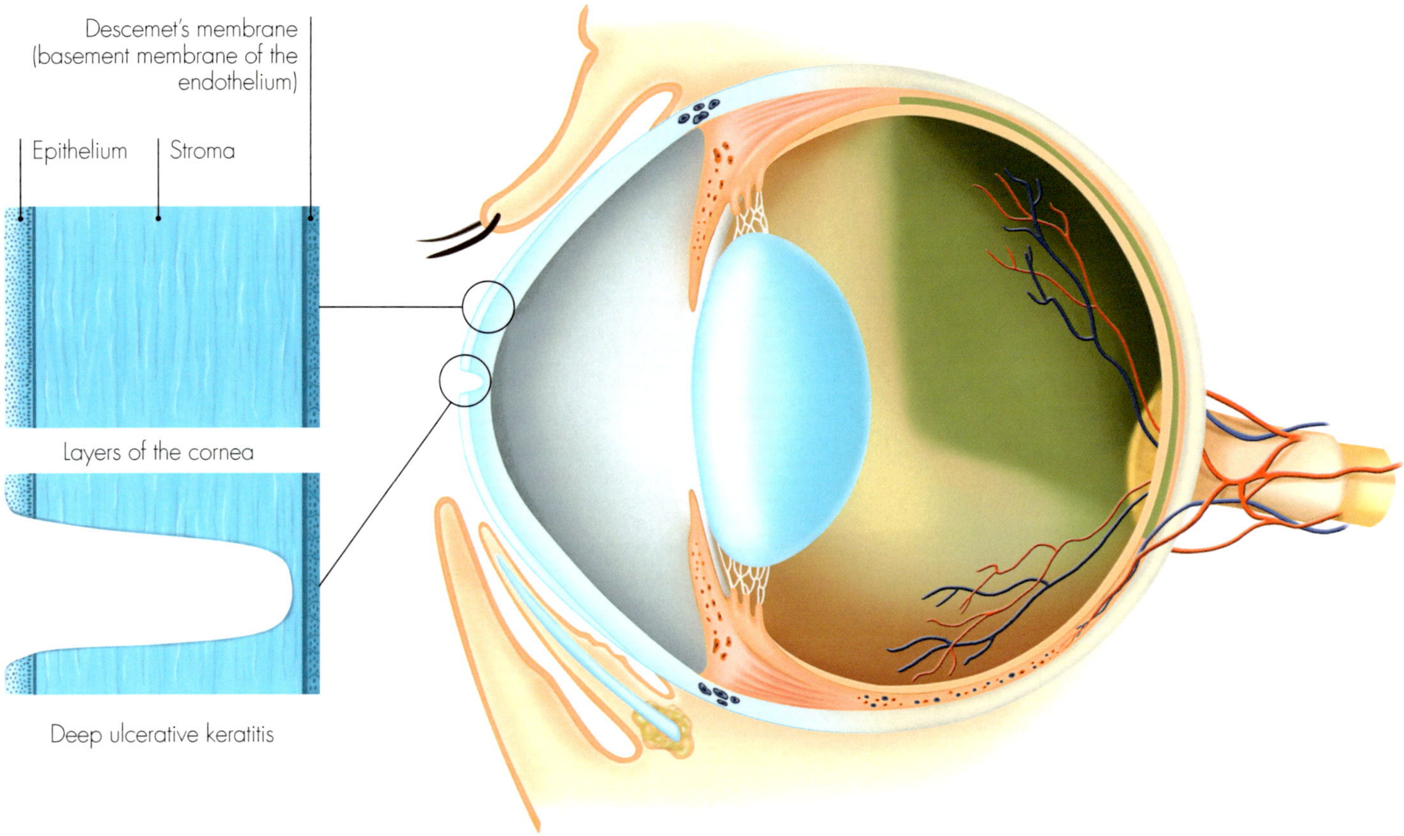

Surgery of deep ulcerative keratitis by means of a conjunctival flap

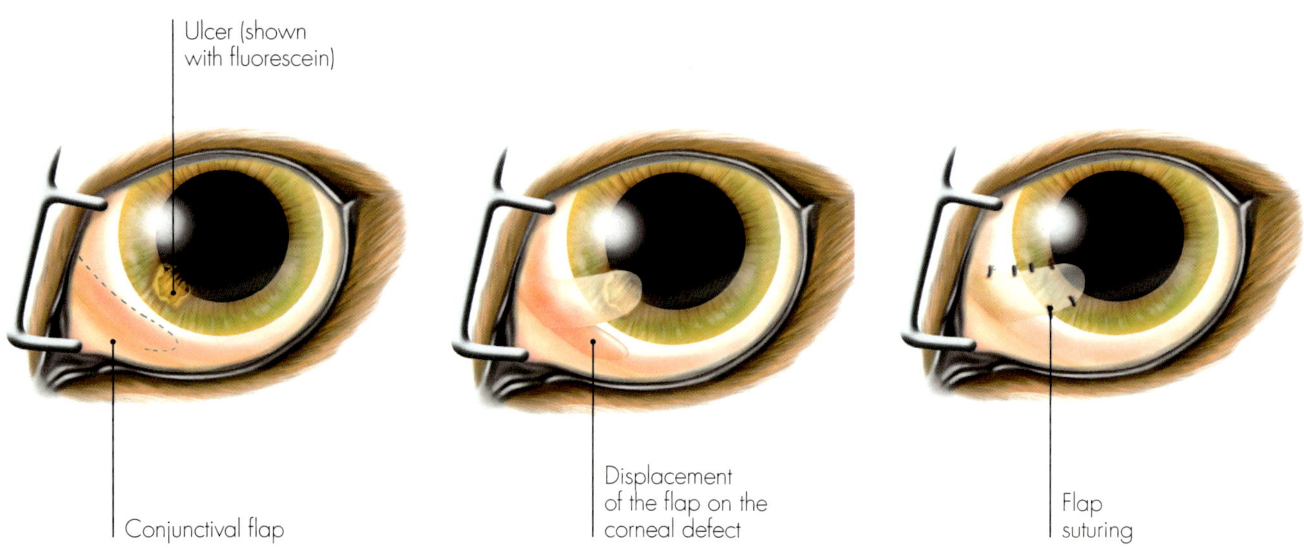

69 Toxoplasmosis

Disease transmissible to humans (zoonosis).

Disease caused by the protozoan *Toxoplasma gondii*. In cats (definitive hosts), the parasite goes through an enteroepithelial cycle. Oocysts are released in the faeces and become infective in the exterior environment. The severity of the clinical picture depends on the affected organ, on the degree of necrosis (cell death) and on the type of strain of *Toxoplasma gondii*.

Appearance of clinical signs

- After consuming contaminated raw meat or contaminated water.
- In kittens, after birth or during lactation if the mother is infected.
- After reactivation in cats with latent disease.

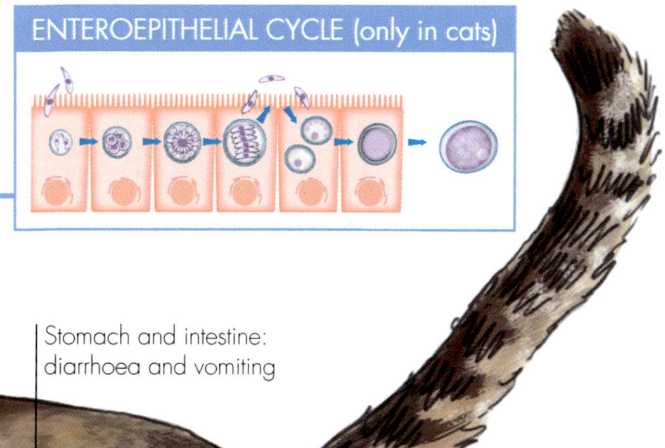

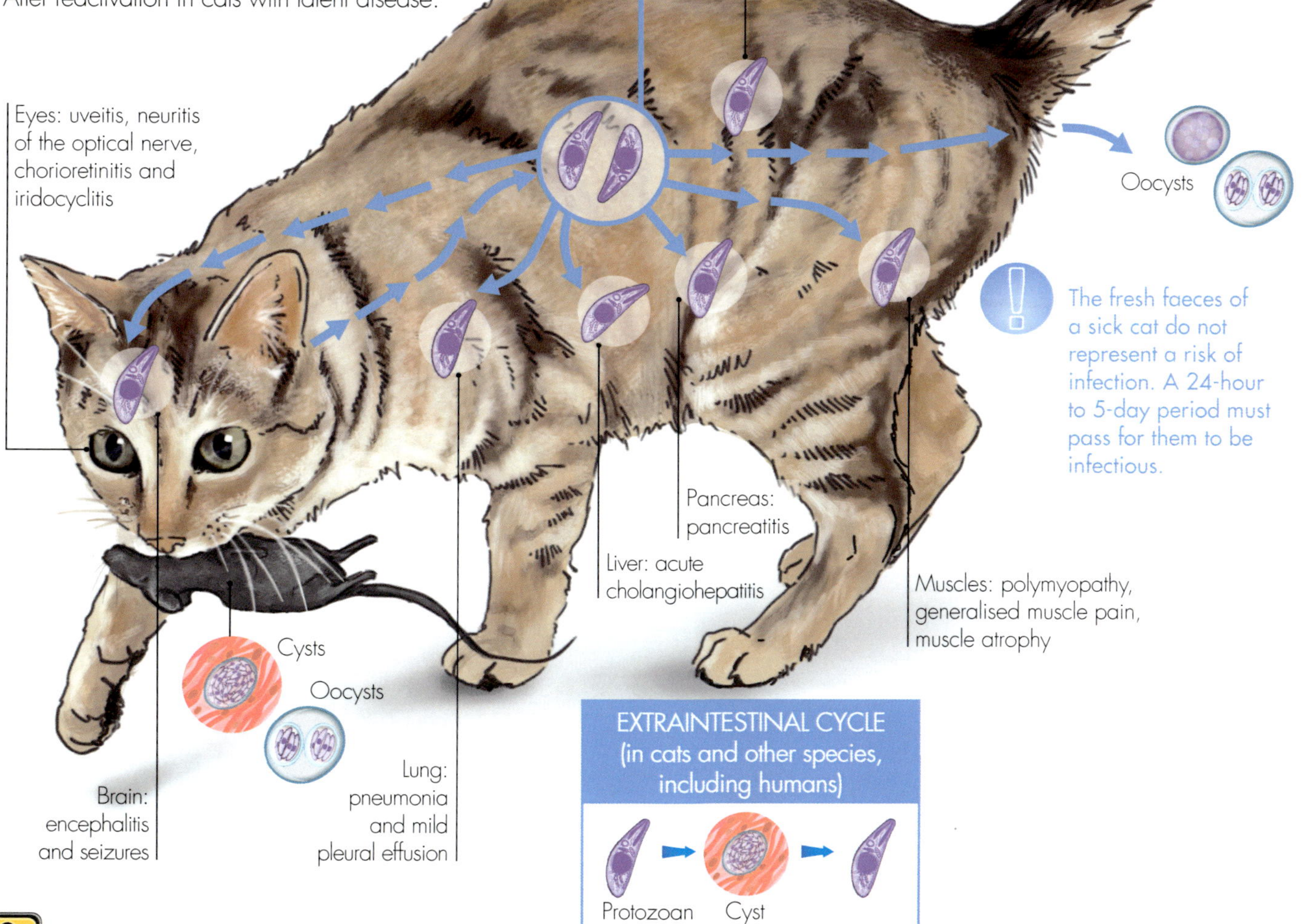

The fresh faeces of a sick cat do not represent a risk of infection. A 24-hour to 5-day period must pass for them to be infectious.

Recommendations

To avoid infection, pregnant women and other people should:

- Eat meat cooked at high temperatures.
- Eat rare-cooked meat only if it has previously been frozen for two days.
- Wash their hands after gardening or cooking.
- Not drink untreated water.
- Clean the cat's litter trays daily, using a shovel and washing hands afterwards.

70 Feline infectious peritonitis (FIP)

Caused by feline coronavirus (FCoV), which is spread through faeces. FCoV infection causes few digestive signs, but 5–10 % of infected cats will develop feline infectious peritonitis (FIP), a progressive disease that is associated with very high mortality and mainly affects young cats in shelters or catteries.

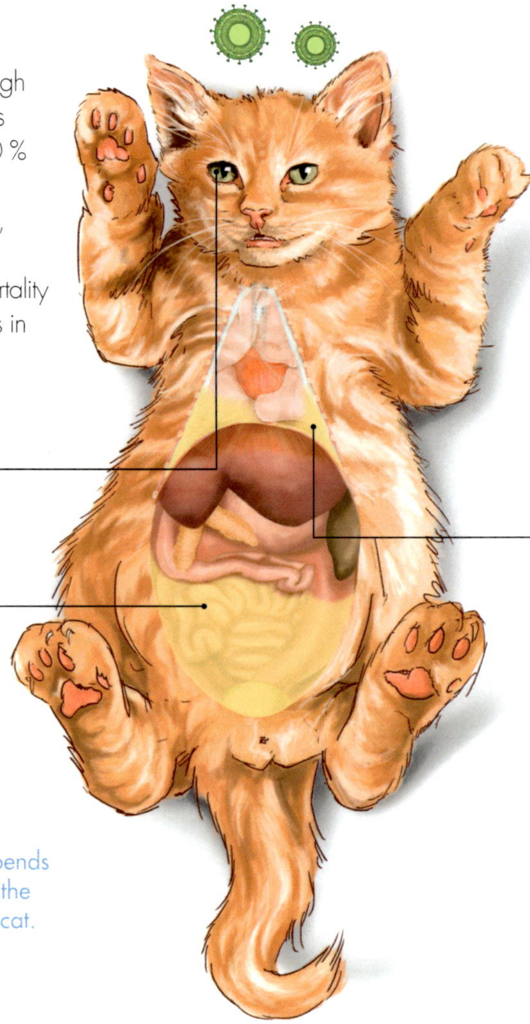

Risk factors

- Groups of cats (shared litter tray).
- Age: cats under one year of age are the most affected.
- Associated infections (bacteria, parasites, other viruses).
- Poor hygiene, overcrowding.

Clinical signs

Common signs in both the dry and wet forms:

- Fever with no response to antibiotic treatment.
- Depression.
- Progressive loss of weight.
- Growth problems in kittens.

The progression of the disease depends on the interaction of the virus with the immune system of each individual cat.

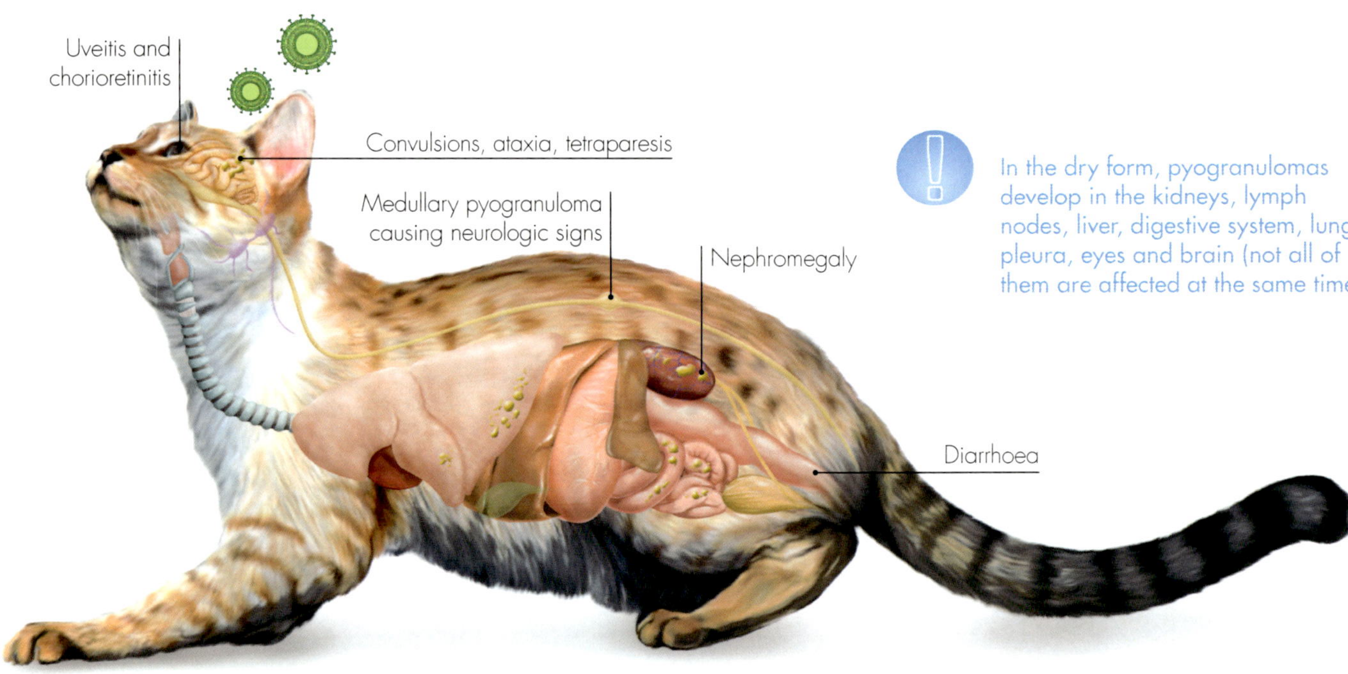

In the dry form, pyogranulomas develop in the kidneys, lymph nodes, liver, digestive system, lungs, pleura, eyes and brain (not all of them are affected at the same time).

71 Feline leukaemia (FeLV)

Feline leukaemia virus is transmitted mainly by saliva, and requires close and prolonged contact between cats. Less frequently it is transmitted by nasal discharge, tears, faeces, urine, milk, semen, vaginal fluids, and the placenta.

Vaccination should start at 8–9 weeks of age, with a second dose administered 3–4 weeks later. Cats should be vaccinated again 1 year later and subsequently according to their level of risk.

Diagnosis of feline leukaemia is complex. Tests such as ELISA and PCR may be required using both blood and bone marrow samples.

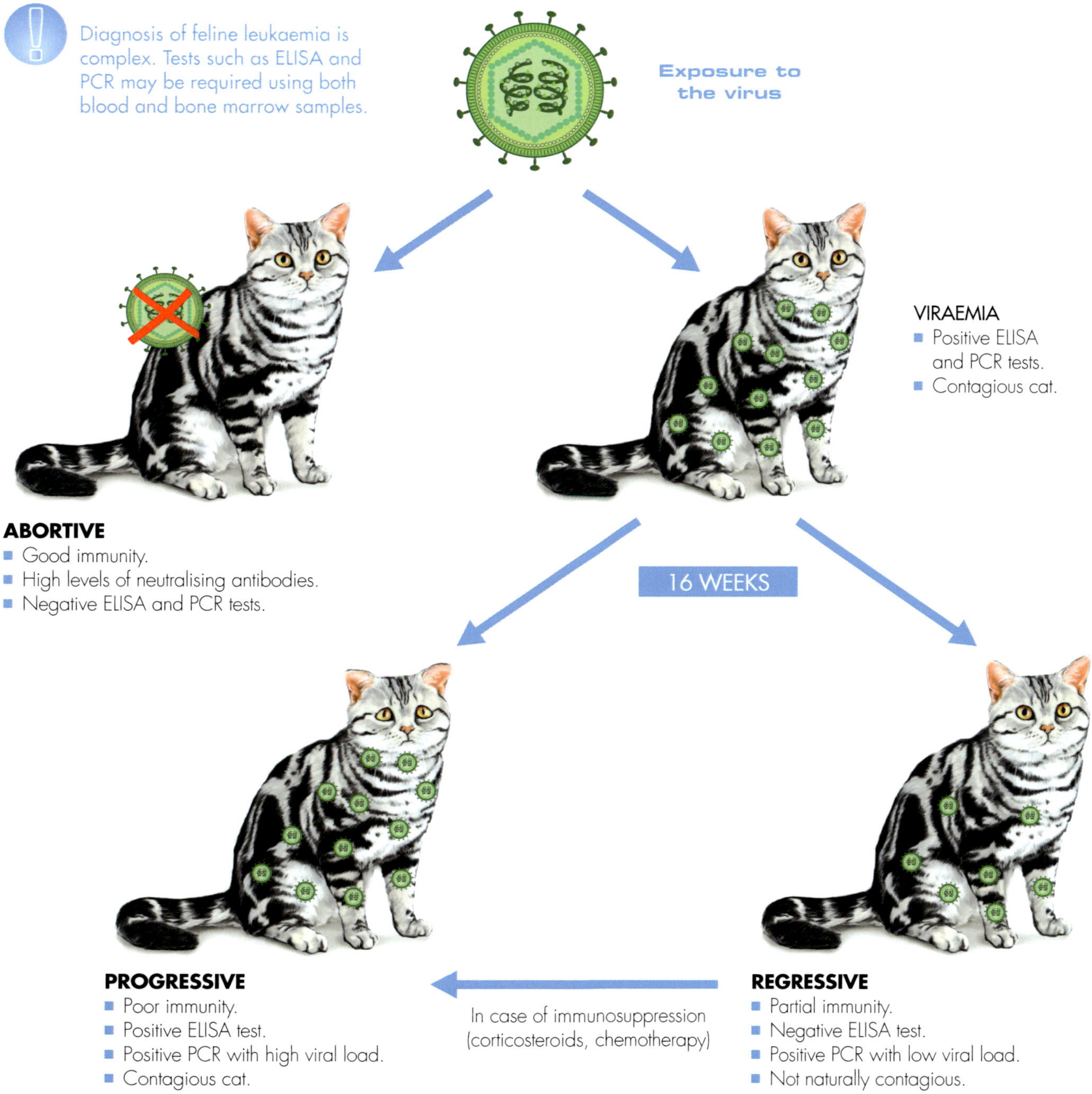

Medical treatment

Currently there is no curative treatment available. However, clinical signs can be alleviated and life expectancy prolonged.

72 Feline immunodeficiency (FIV)

This viral infection is essentially transmitted through saliva or blood in cases of bites.
An infected mother may transmit it to 50 % of her offspring during gestation and lactation.

A blood test (ELISA) must be carried out 15 days and 2 months after the cat has been bitten.

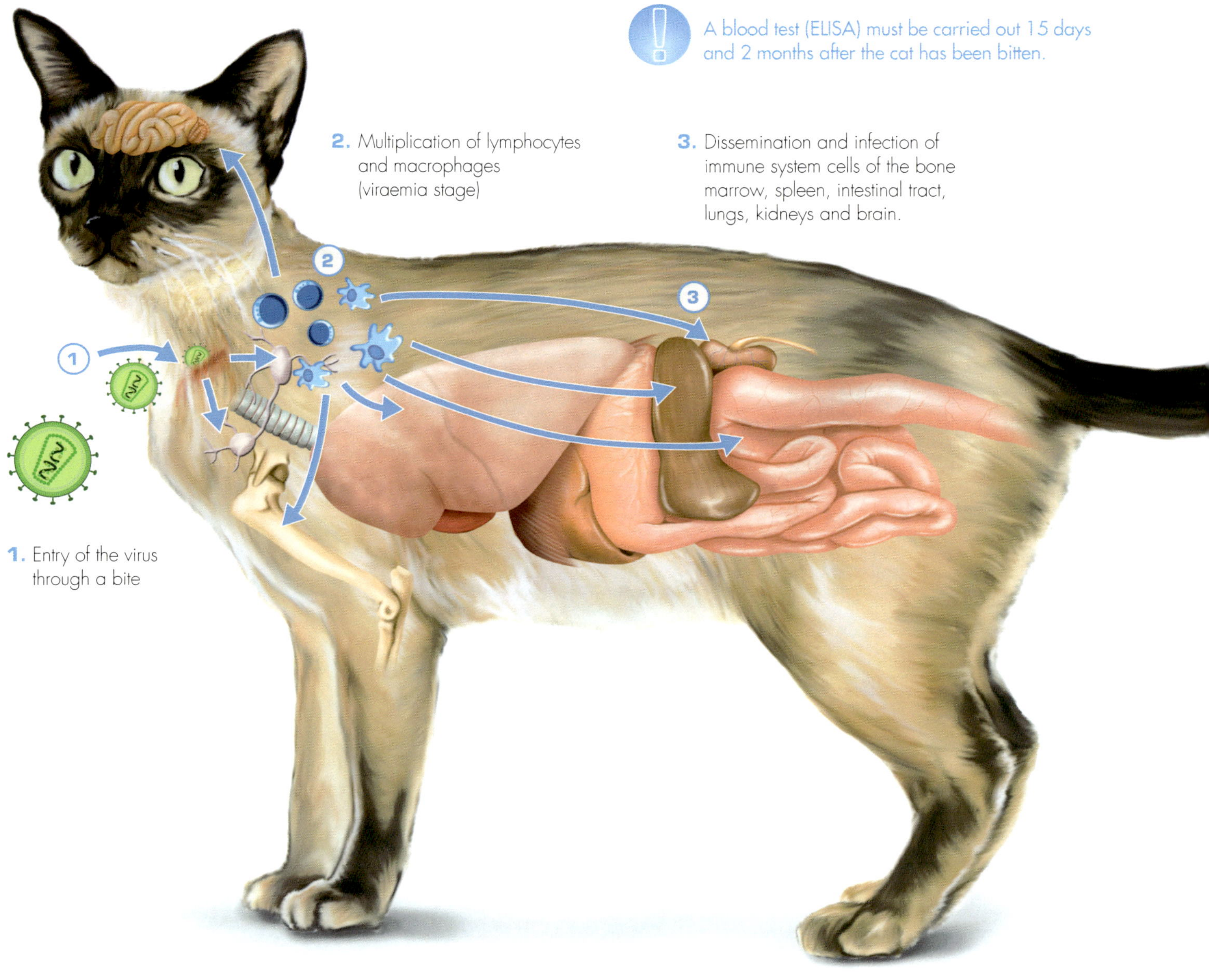

Clinical signs

- When the infection occurs: fever, enlargement of the lymph nodes, apathy and anorexia.
- This is followed by an asymptomatic period that may last for years.
- When the immune system is weakened, an immune-deficiency stage (AIDS) that lasts for several months appears: fever, anorexia, lymph node enlargement, secondary infections (diarrhoea, otitis, conjunctivitis, rhinitis, cutaneous abscesses), gingivostomatitis, immune-mediated anaemia, neurological disorders and tumours.

Diagnosis

- Detection of antibodies in blood in cats >6 months (ELISA) and PCR in cats <6 months.
- Any positive result should be confirmed by a PCR test.

73 Feline panleukopaenia

Disease caused by a parvovirus. Some variants of canine parvoviruses may affect cats. Infection occurs through direct contact with secretions of a sick cat (faeces, saliva, etc.) or with a contaminated environment.

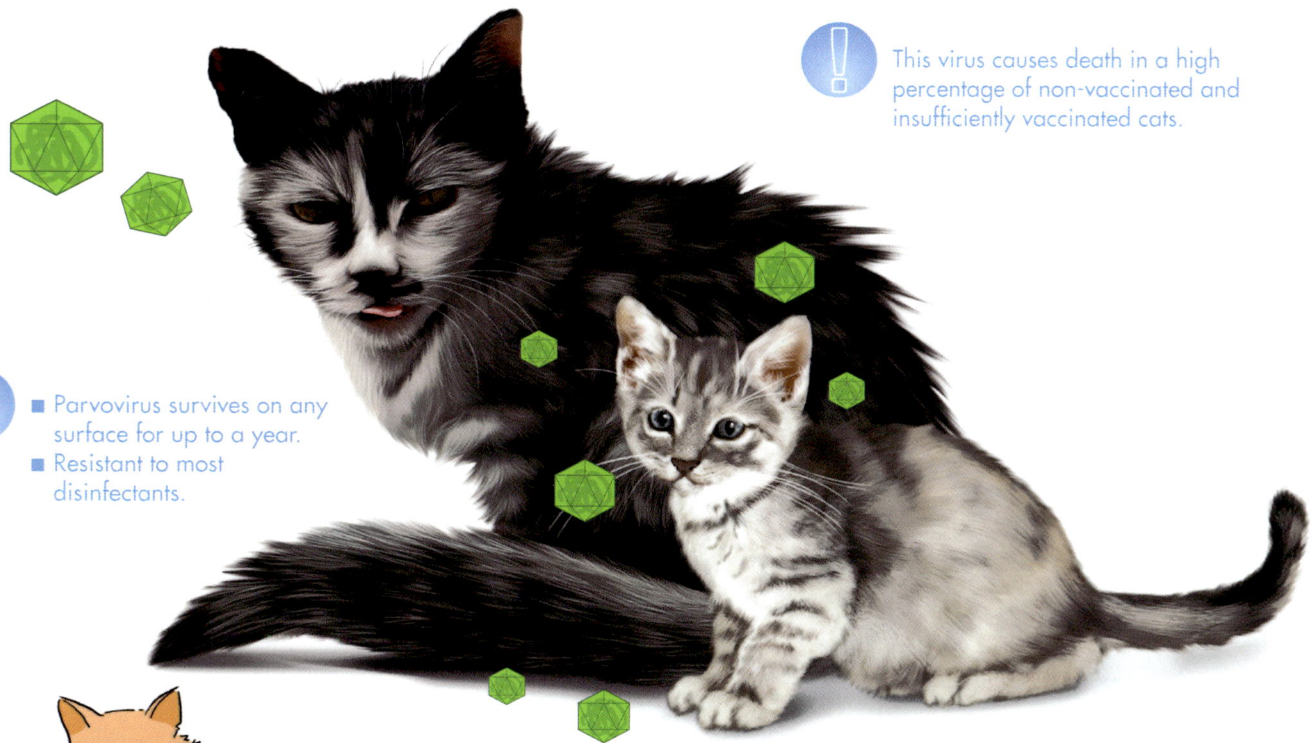

This virus causes death in a high percentage of non-vaccinated and insufficiently vaccinated cats.

- Parvovirus survives on any surface for up to a year.
- Resistant to most disinfectants.

In pregnant females

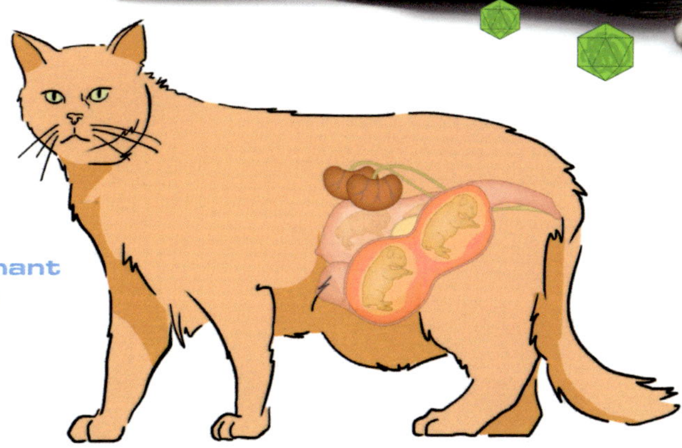

GESTATION (2 MONTHS)		
Early infection	Mid-gestation infection	Late infection
Foetal death and resorption	Abortions and foetal mummification	Birth of kittens with lesions in the brain and cerebellum

Clinical signs

They occur between 5 and 14 days after exposure to the virus:

- Fever, intense depression.
- Anorexia, vomiting.
- Sepsis with haemorrhagic diarrhoea and jaundice.
- Sudden death in cats of up to 1 year of age.

Recommendations

- Disinfect all the areas in contact with the sick cat with bleach diluted at 1:30 for 10 minutes.
- Only correctly vaccinated cats should enter the areas that could not be appropriately cleaned.

All the cats should be vaccinated, even indoor cats due to the risk of infection through shoes, clothes, etc.

74 Feline herpesvirus

Type I feline herpesvirus is the causative agent of feline rhinotracheitis. This virus is capable of multiplying in cells of the ocular conjunctiva, the respiratory system, and neurons. Multiplication in neurons causes it to remain **latent** for life after acute infection, and to subsequently **reactivate** during processes that cause immune suppression.

It is one of the main agents responsible for the feline respiratory disease complex, together with calicivirus, *Bordetella bronchiseptica*, *Chlamydophila felis* and *Mycoplasma* spp.

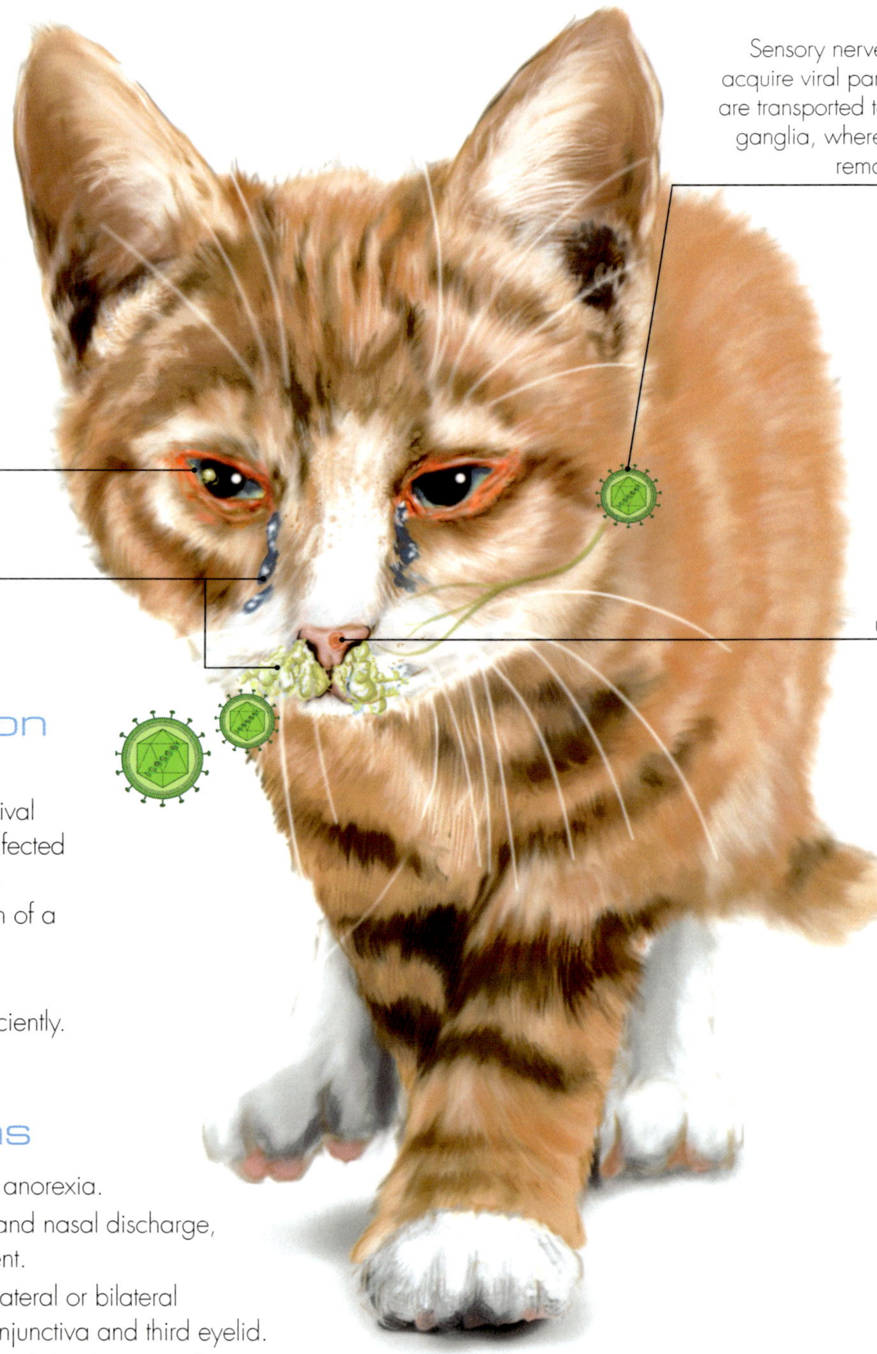
Sensory nerve endings acquire viral particles that are transported to sensory ganglia, where the virus remains latent
Corneal ulcer
Abundant ocular and nasal discharge
Skin ulceration

Transmission

- By direct contact with oronasal and conjunctival secretions of acutely infected cats or those that have undergone reactivation of a latent infection.
- Via human hands and objects, albeit less efficiently.

Clinical signs

- Fever, depression and anorexia.
- Rhinitis with sneezing and nasal discharge, which becomes purulent.
- Ocular discharge, unilateral or bilateral inflammation of the conjunctiva and third eyelid.
- Corneal inflammation and development of superficial corneal ulcers that may evolve to deep corneal ulcers and even corneal sequestra.
- Uncommon: ulcers in the mouth, hypersalivation, cough and facial ulcers.

Almost 80 % of cats infected by the herpesvirus become carriers for the rest of their lives. Stress and immunosuppressive treatments may reactivate it. Cats should be vaccinated against herpesvirus based on their level of risk.

75 Feline calicivirus

It is a very infectious virus that is widespread among cats. It can be transmitted through saliva, tears, nasal secretions, faeces and urine of sick animals or chronic carriers of the virus. Our hands and objects are another source of infection.

Acute presentation

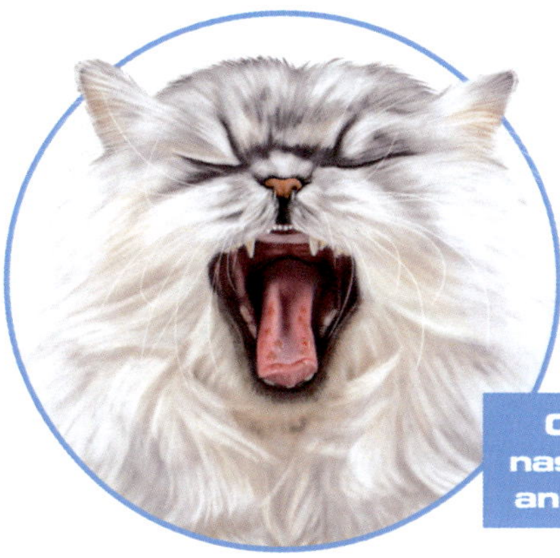

Oral ulcers, nasal discharge and pneumonia

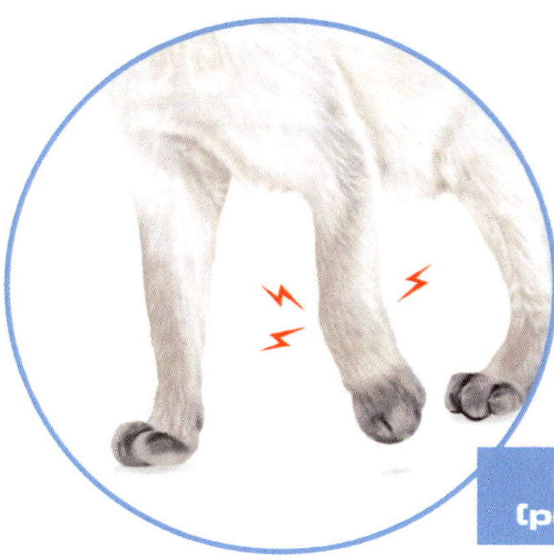

Lameness (polyarthritis)

After the acute presentation, the virus is completely eliminated within approximately 1 month, although some cats continue to be carriers.

More virulent strains

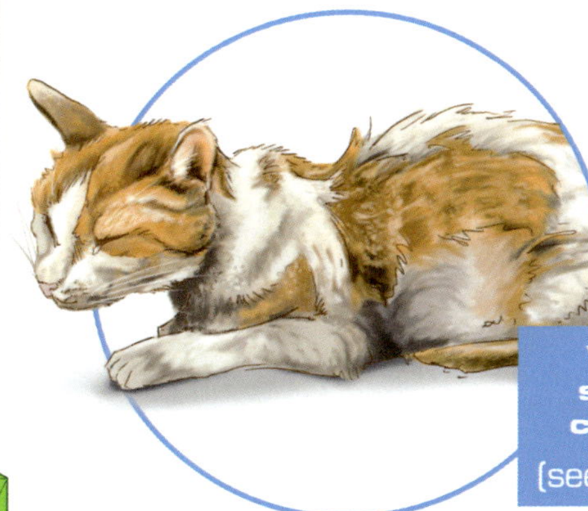

Virulent systemic calicivirus (see next sheet)

Chronic presentation

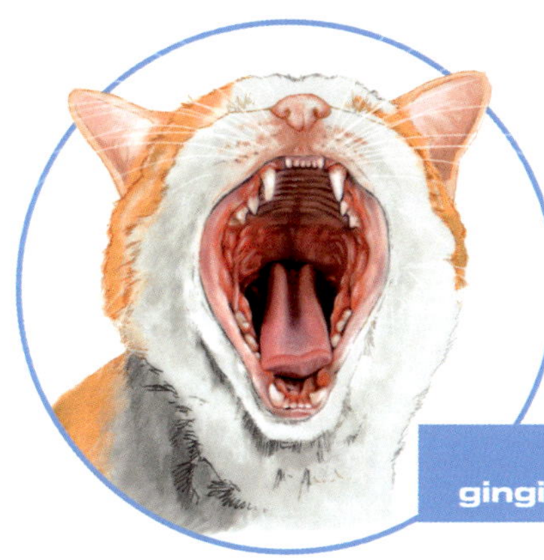

Chronic gingivostomatitis

Vaccines do not prevent the animal from being infected, but are very effective to reduce the severity of the clinical signs.

Recommendations

- The environment can be disinfected with sodium hypochlorite (bleach) diluted at 1:32 in water.
- Hands can be disinfected with 70 % ethanol.

Clinical signs

They depend on the type of strain and its virulence:

- Acute infection:
  - Acute oral and upper airway disease, with fever, oral ulcers, sneezing and nasal discharge.
  - Polyarthritis: transient lameness with fever.
  - Systemic virulent calicivirus syndrome.
- Chronic infection:
  - Chronic gingivostomatitis (see sheet no. 57).

76 Systemic virulent calicivirus

Feline calicivirus can give rise to a more serious syndrome known as **virulent systemic feline calicivirus**, which is caused by a more virulent mutation of this feline virus that occurs in communities.

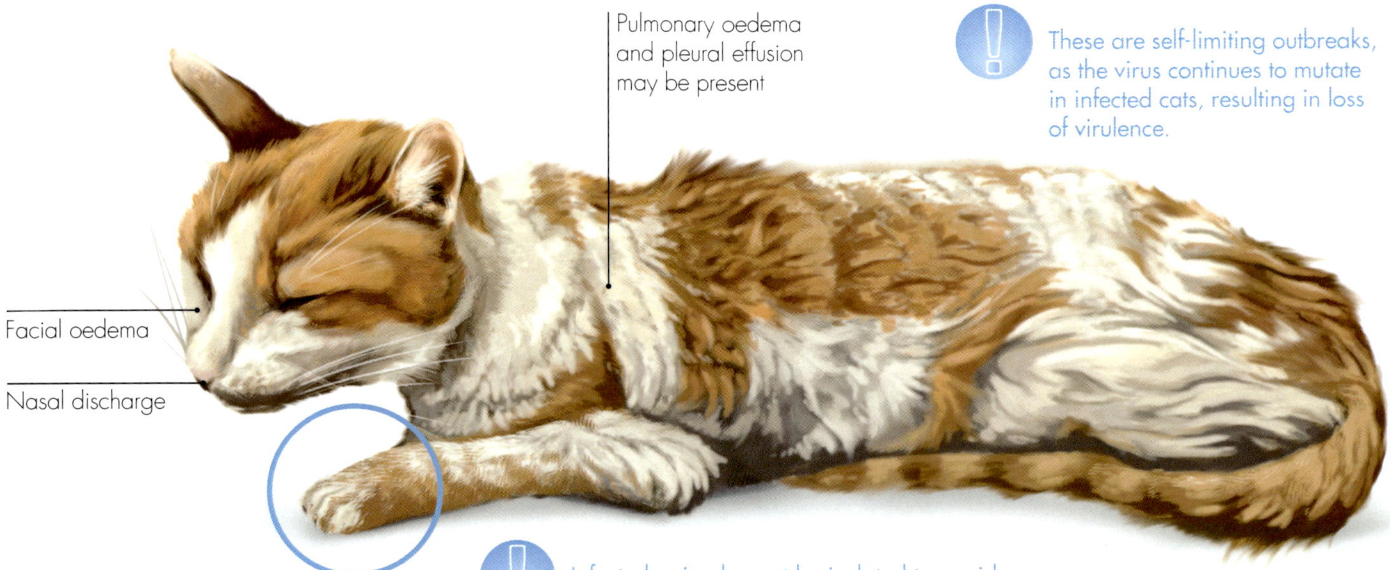
Pulmonary oedema and pleural effusion may be present
Facial oedema
Nasal discharge

These are self-limiting outbreaks, as the virus continues to mutate in infected cats, resulting in loss of virulence.

Infected animals must be isolated to avoid contagion of other cats, as vaccinated animals can also be infected.

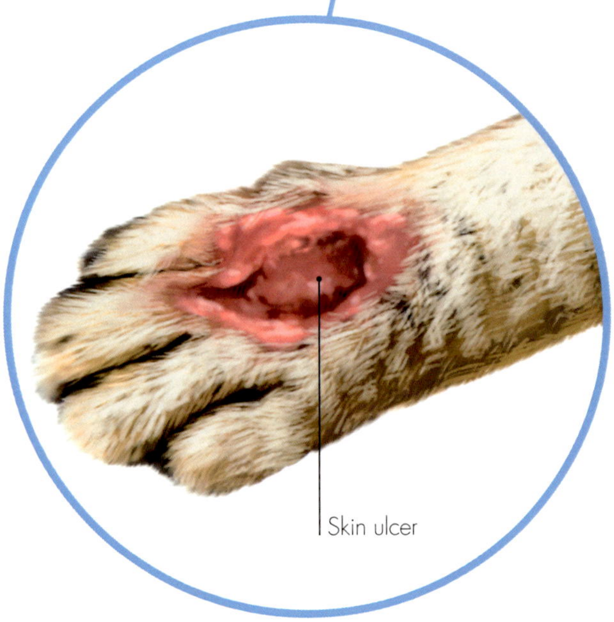

Clinical signs

- Signs appear 1–12 days after exposure. The clinical presentation is more severe in adult cats, with a mortality rate of up to 67 %.
- Initial signs are typical of feline calicivirus, and consist of upper respiratory signs, oral ulcers, and fever.
- These progress to the development of vasculitis with the appearance of:
  - Ulceration and skin necrosis.
  - Facial and limb oedema.
  - Multisystem failure with jaundice due to liver necrosis, pulmonary oedema or pneumonia, disseminated intravascular coagulation (DIC), ascites, and pleural effusion.

Diagnosis

Based on clinical signs and PCR of tissue samples.

Surfaces must be disinfected with 5 % sodium hypochlorite solution.

Treatment

- Fluid therapy, analgesia, and broad-spectrum antibiotics to treat respiratory and oral infections.
- Administration of corticosteroids and feline omega interferon has also been reported.

77 Feline chlamydiosis

The disease is caused by *Chlamidophyla felis* bacteria. Infection occurs through contact with conjunctival, nasal and vaginal secretions as well as through faeces. Our hands and objects (food and water bowls) may be a route of infection.

Newborn cats become infected through their mother's genital mucosa and develop severe conjunctivitis short after birth. Cats >1 year of age run a lower risk of becoming infected as they develop immunity.

Vaccination does not completely protect against infection, but significantly reduces clinical signs. It is recommended in cats living in groups.

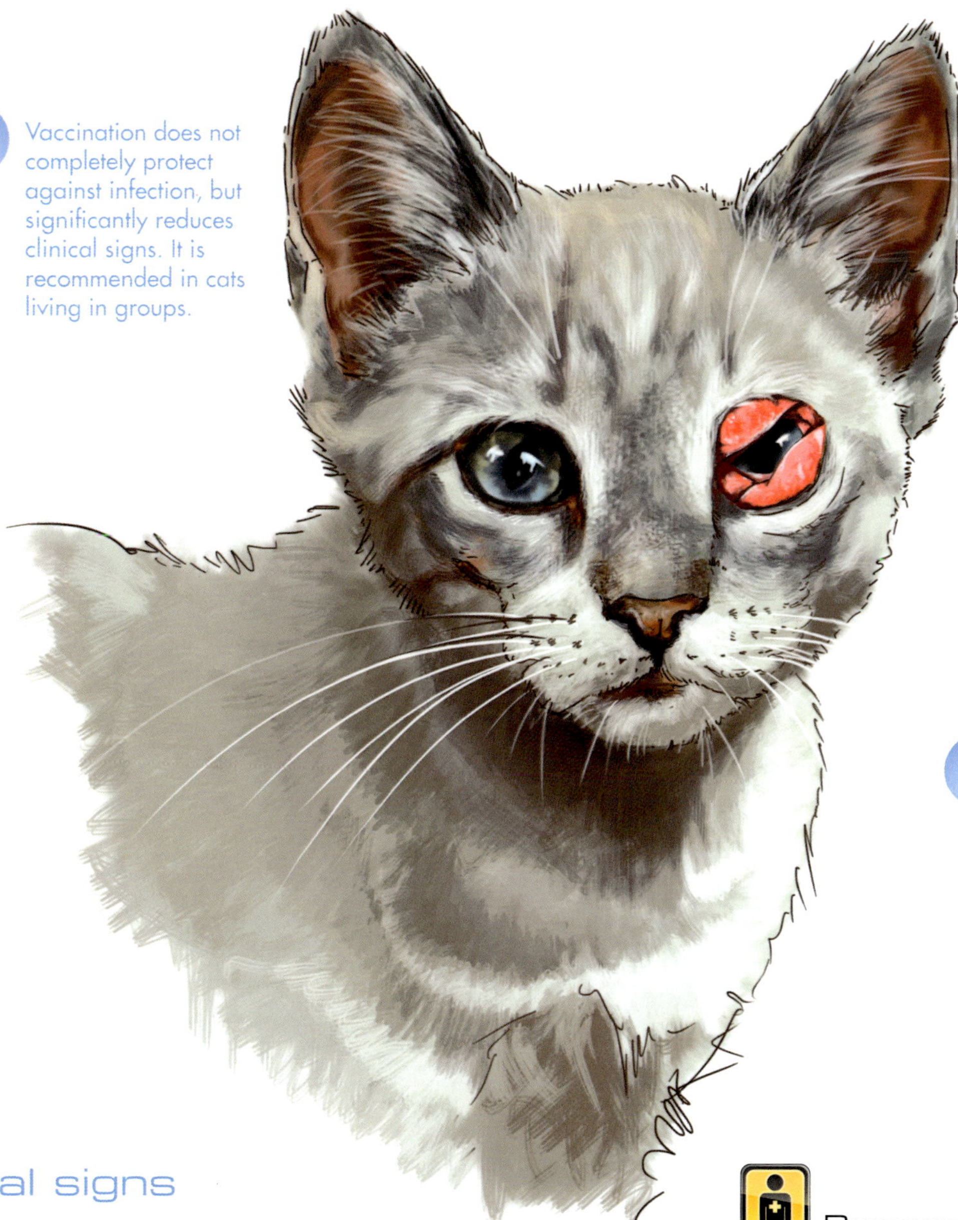

Conditions such as overcrowding, lack of hygiene, stress and poor ventilation favour reinfections.

Clinical signs

- Severe conjunctivitis and persisting tearing (watery or thick and purulent tears). Infection is initially unilateral, and then affects the other eye.
- Inflamed and half-closed eyes (blepharospasm).
- Uncommon: sneezing, nasal discharge and fever.

Recommendations

- The environment can be disinfected with sodium hypochlorite (bleach) diluted at 1:32 in water (these bacteria only survive for a few days in the environment).
- Hands can be disinfected with 70 % ethanol.

78 Feeding tubes

Indications

- Hepatic lipidosis.
- Anorexia caused by any disease accompanied by a loss of 20 % of the animal's weight.
- Facial trauma.
- Oral surgeries.

! These systems give good results and are a better alternative to force feeding, since this latter option can lead to an aversion syndrome, which will result in the cat needing more time to eat by itself again.

Feeding tube by means of oesophagostomy

Advantages

- Does not require an Elizabethan collar.
- Does not annoy the animal.
- Can be left for up to 3 months.
- The cat can eat voluntarily at any time.
- Allows the administration of medication through the tube.

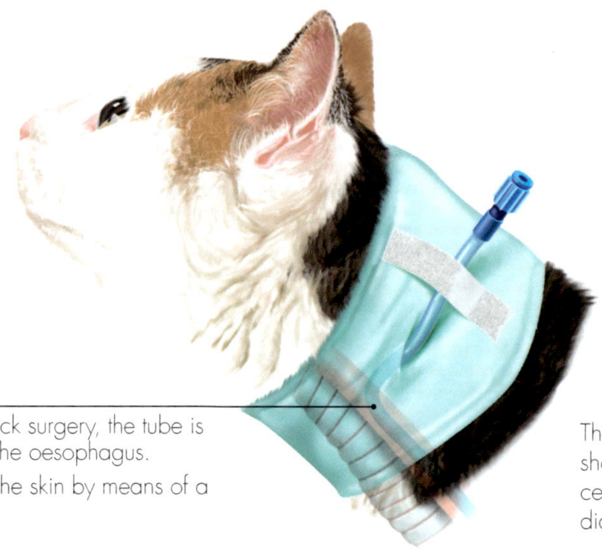

Nasooesophageal tube

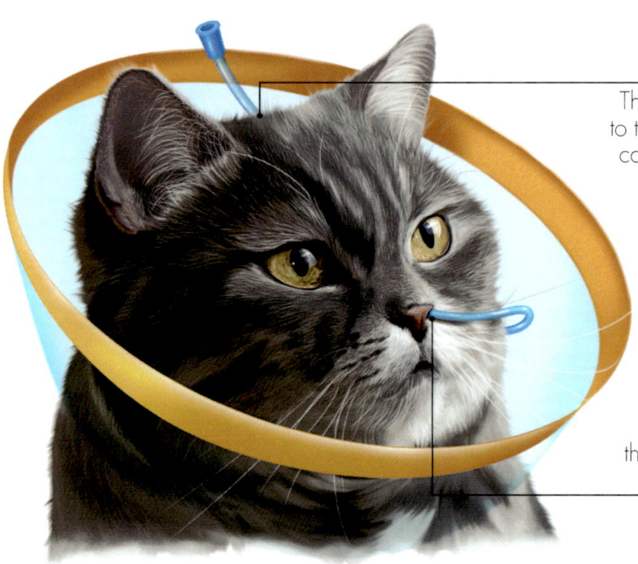
The tube is attached to the cat's head so it can be manipulated
Introduction of the feeding tube into the digestive system through the nose

Advantages

- Simple procedure.

Disadvantages

- Requires an Elizabethan collar.
- Is uncomfortable for the cat.
- Can only be left for 6 days.

79 Bone marrow aspiration technique

Bone marrow is the most important haematopoietic organ (production of blood cells) organ in the organism.

Aspiration of bone from the head of the humerus

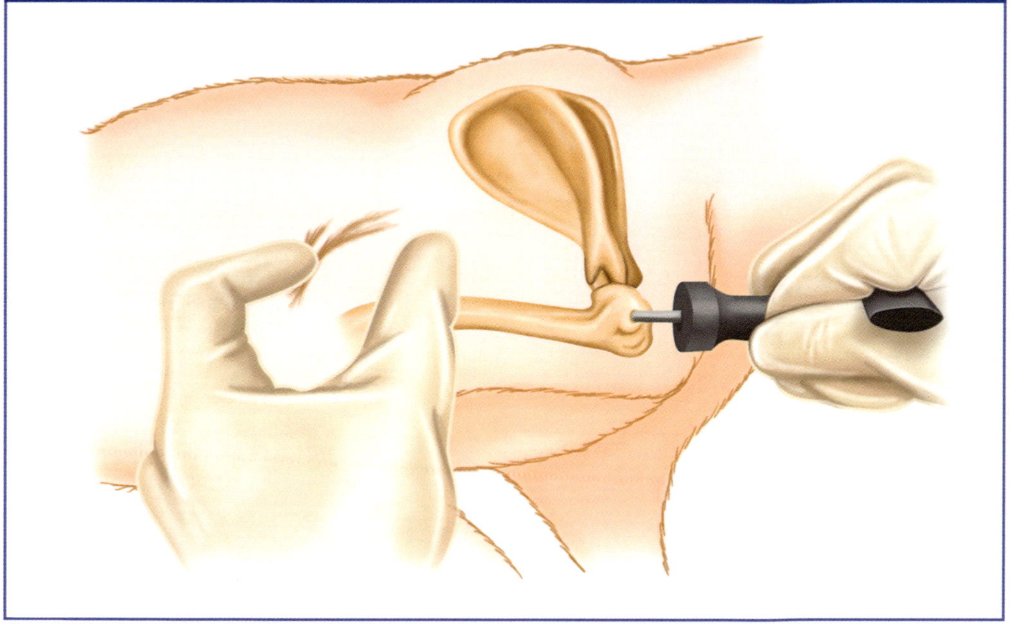

> The aspiration and analysis of bone marrow is useful for the diagnosis of anaemia and infectious diseases such as feline leukaemia.

Aspiration of bone marrow from the iliac crest

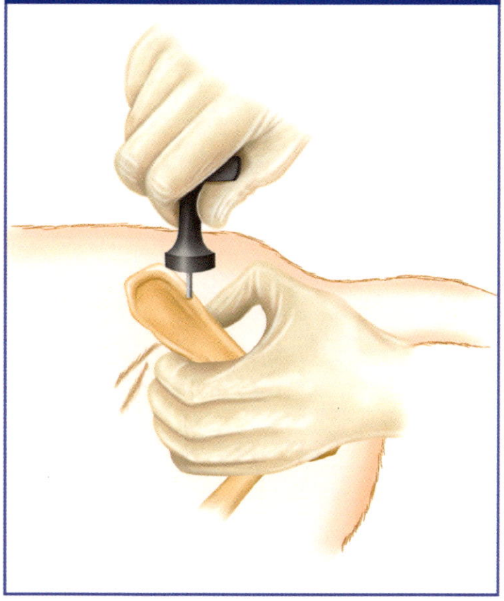

Aspiration of bone marrow from the femur

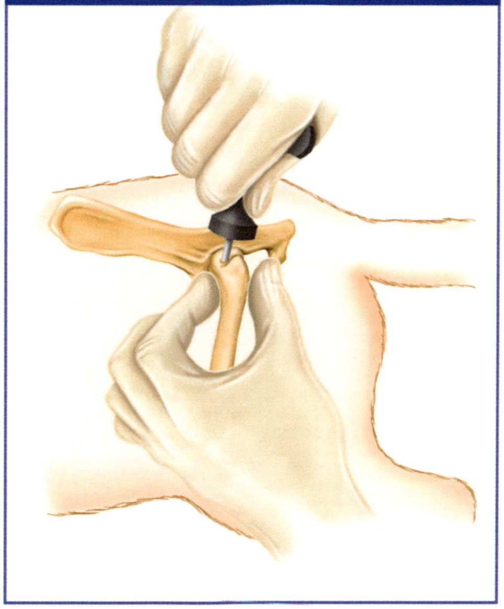

Method

- The bone marrow is gently aspirated using a 10 ml syringe and special bone marrow needles or, in the case of fine-boned cats, 18 G hypodermic needles.
- Smears are prepared for cytology.
- Part of the sample is stored in EDTA for specific tests (feline leukaemia PCR).
- The bones of choice are the head of the humerus, the iliac crest, and the femur.

80 Urethral catheterisation and cystocentesis

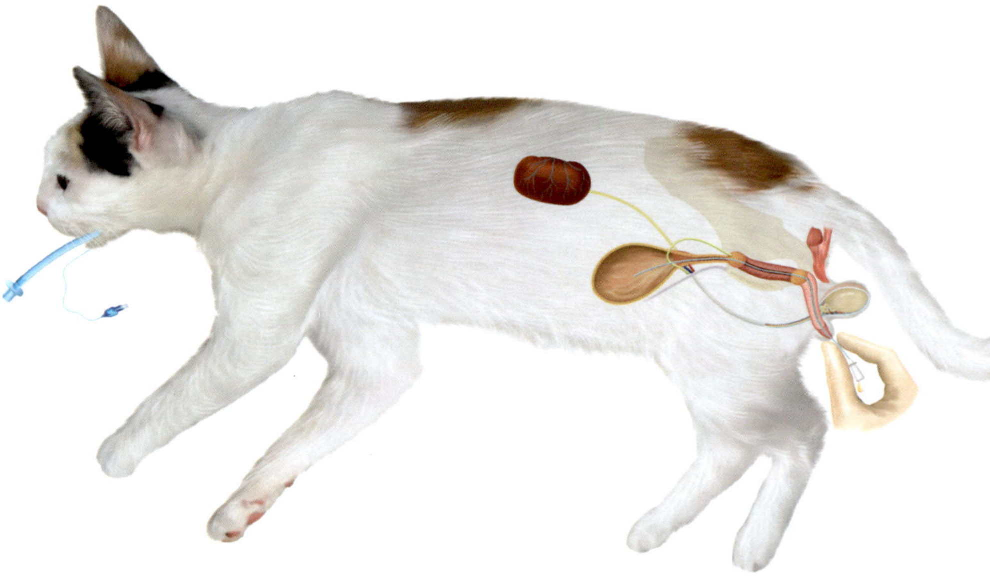

Urethral catheterisation

- This is performed in cases in which urethral obstruction occurs (the cat is unable to urinate).
- It consists of the introduction of a catheter through the penis into the bladder, generally for a maximum of 24–48 hours.
- It always requires anaesthesia and intensive analgesic treatment.

Cystocentesis

- For the diagnosis of urinary infections it is necessary to obtain a sample by cystocentesis.
- This consists of puncturing the bladder with a fine needle.
- It is a painless procedure.
- The urine sample obtained will be sent in sterile conditions for culture and an antibiogram.

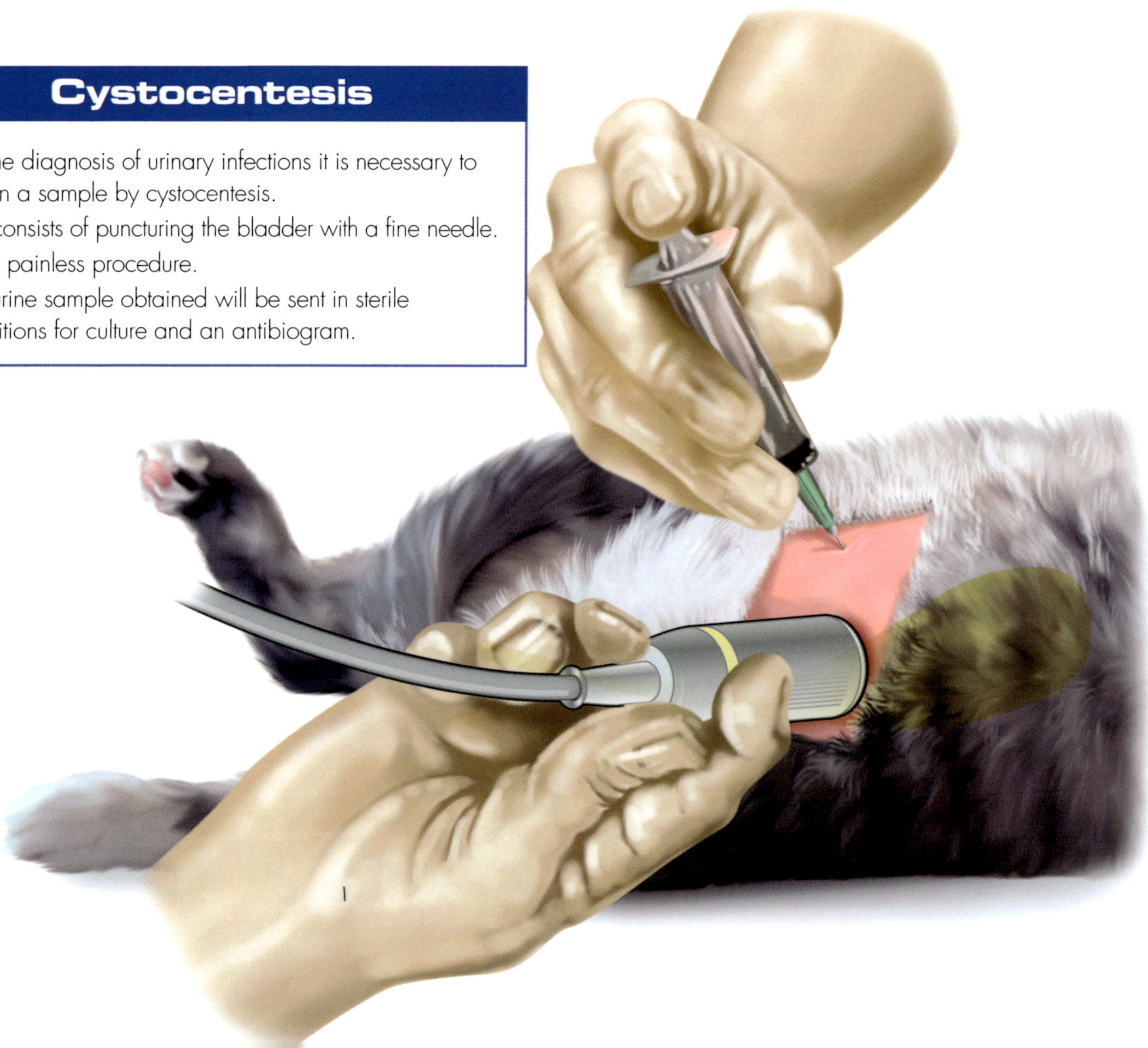

81 Thoracic drainage

Thoracostomy and thoracocentesis

In cases of pyothroax, chylothorax and pneumothorax, the placement of a thoracostomy tube until the process resolver is required.

The accumulation of fluid in the pleural space causes respiratory difficulties. Its removal by means of thoracocentesis allows the diagnosis of the cause and considerably improves the patient's respiratory capacity.

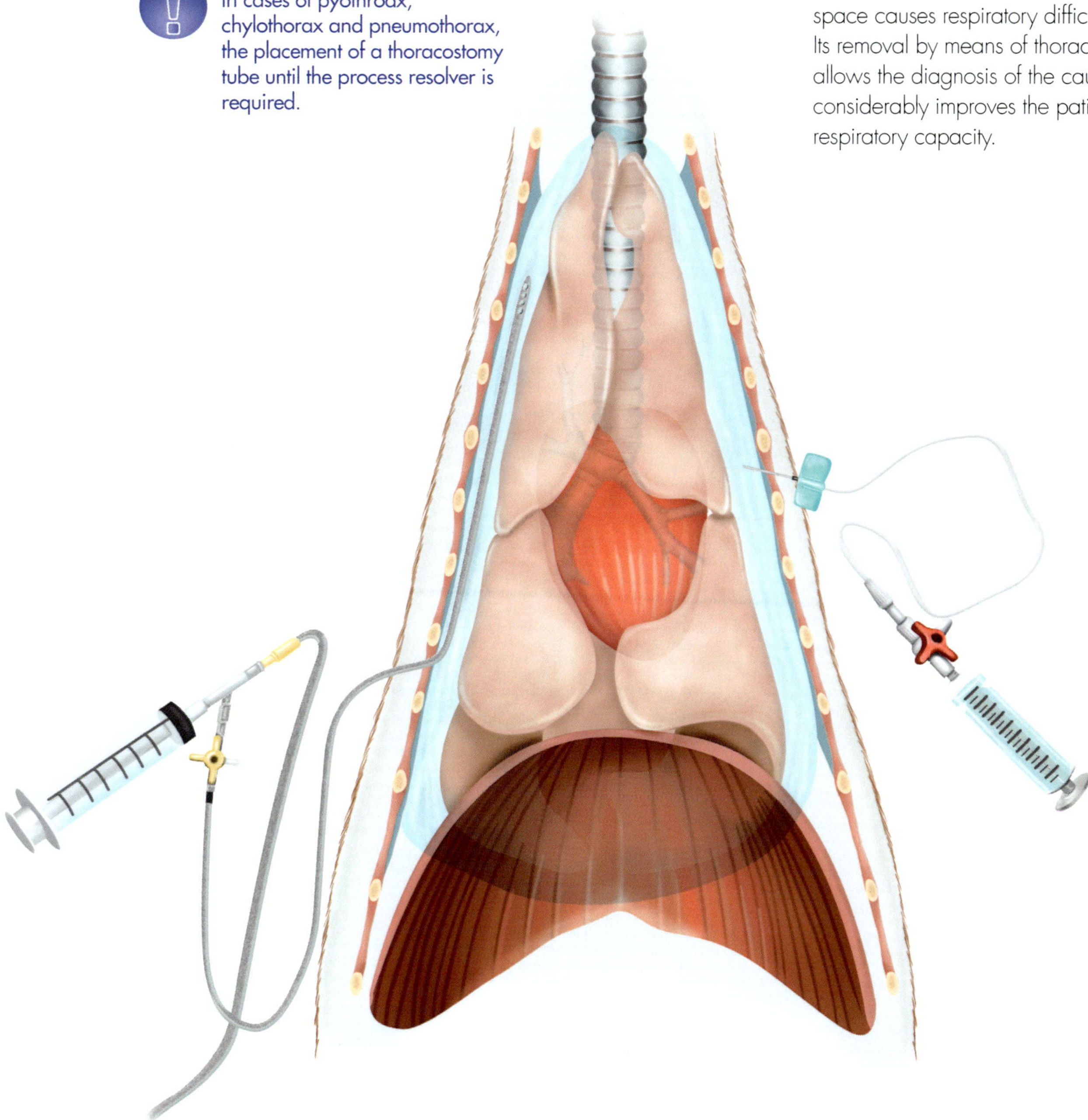

Thoracostomy with a tube

A thoracostomy consists in the placement of a thin tube into the pleural space, which allows the removal of the fluid that is continuously being formed.

Thoracocentesis

Thoracocentesis consists in the removal of accumulated pleural fluid by means of a puncture with a thin needle in the thoracic wall.

82 Collection of cerebrospinal fluid

Atlantooccipital puncture

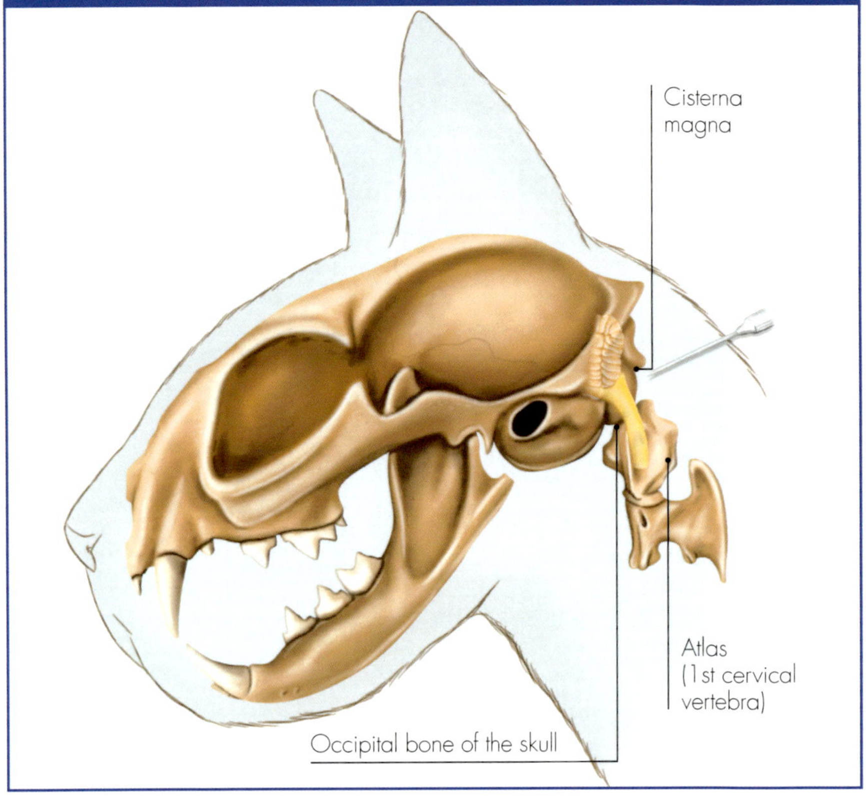

CSF is a colourless fluid which is distributed around the brain and spinal cord.
On occasions, its analysis is necessary to reach a precise diagnosis of the patient's disease: neurological processes of the central nervous system, bacterial infections or infectious diseases.

Technique for CSF collection

- The cat will be anaesthetised, since it must remain completely immobile during the procedure.
- CSF can be collected by means of an atlantooccipital puncture or lumbar puncture (between L5–L6 and L6–L7).

Lumbar puncture

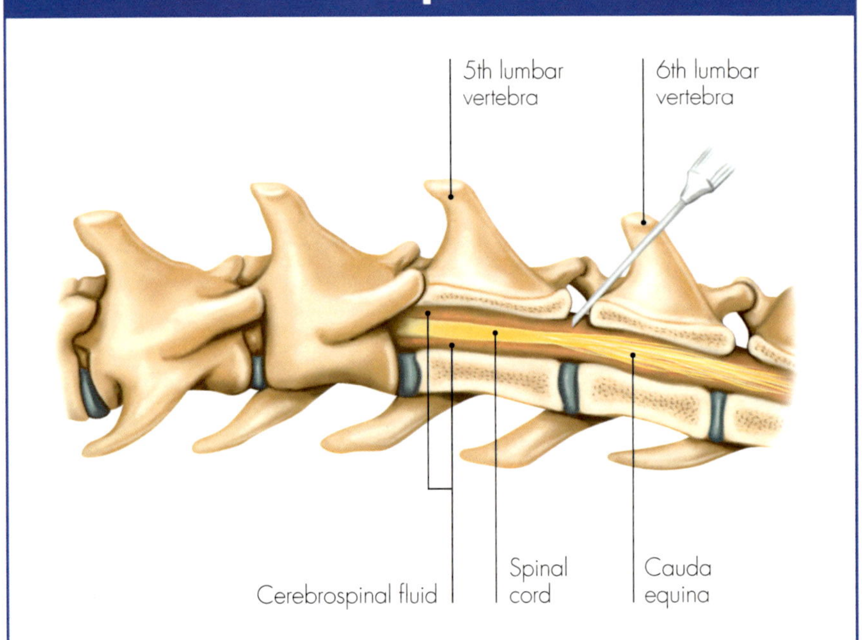

CSF analyses and cultures determine its cellular composition, biochemical characteristics and the possible presence of infectious agents.

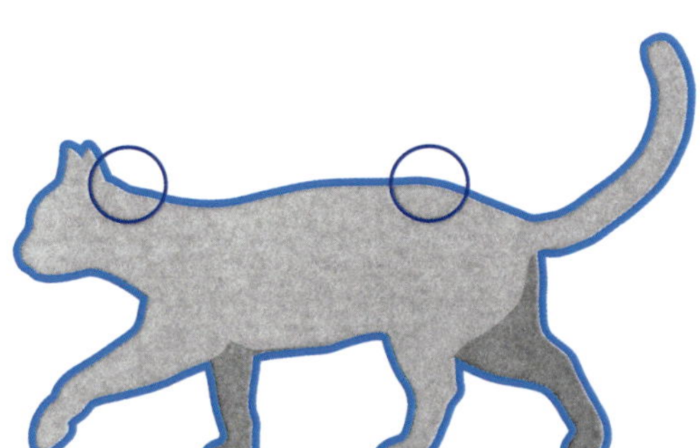

83 How to administer drugs

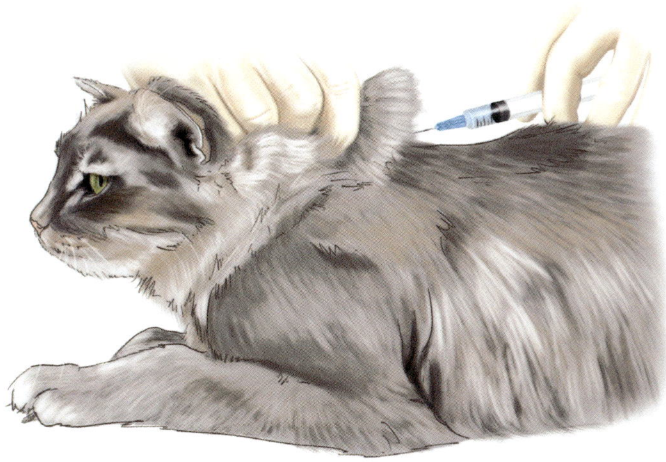

Subcutaneous injection

Eye drops

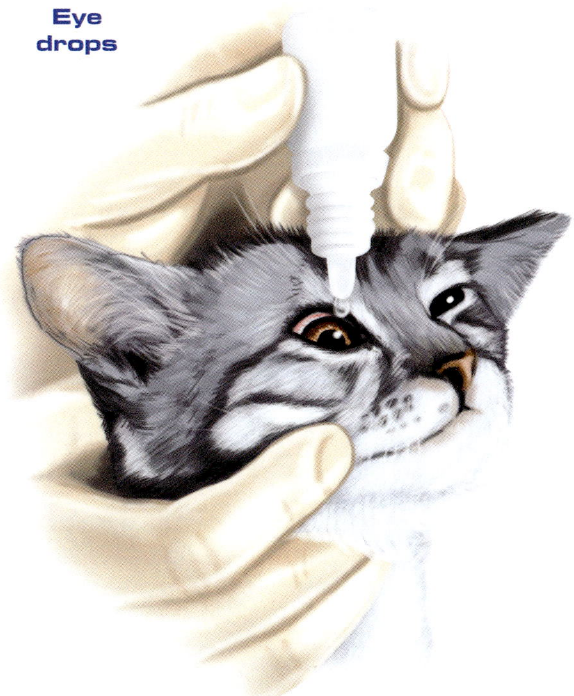

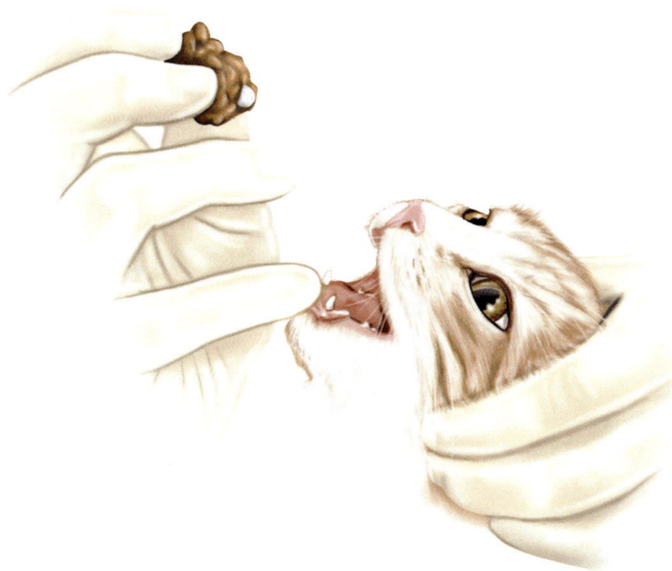

Drugs should never be mixed with the cat's usual food, as the cat would hate it from that moment on.

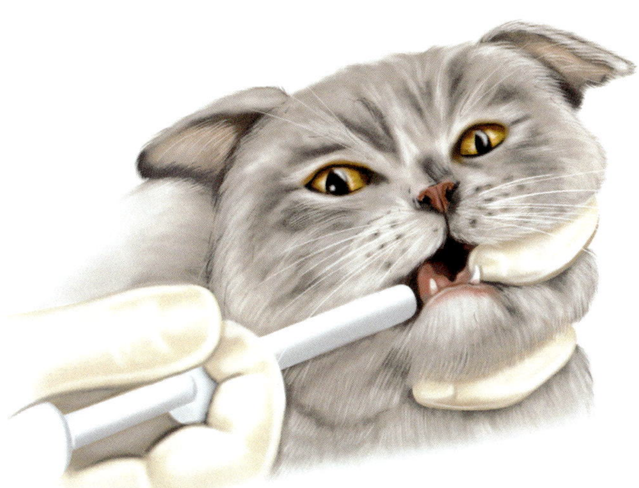

Administration of drugs by oral route

- The pill can be wrapped in meat, bread or butter to hide its taste.
- Water should always be given with a syringe immediately after administering drugs such as doxycycline or clyndamycin.
- The pills can be crushed and administered with water or sweet milk (if the veterinary surgeon considers it necessary).
- It is possible to use a pill gun instead of a syringe.

84 Postures and expressions in cats

Aggressive postures in cats

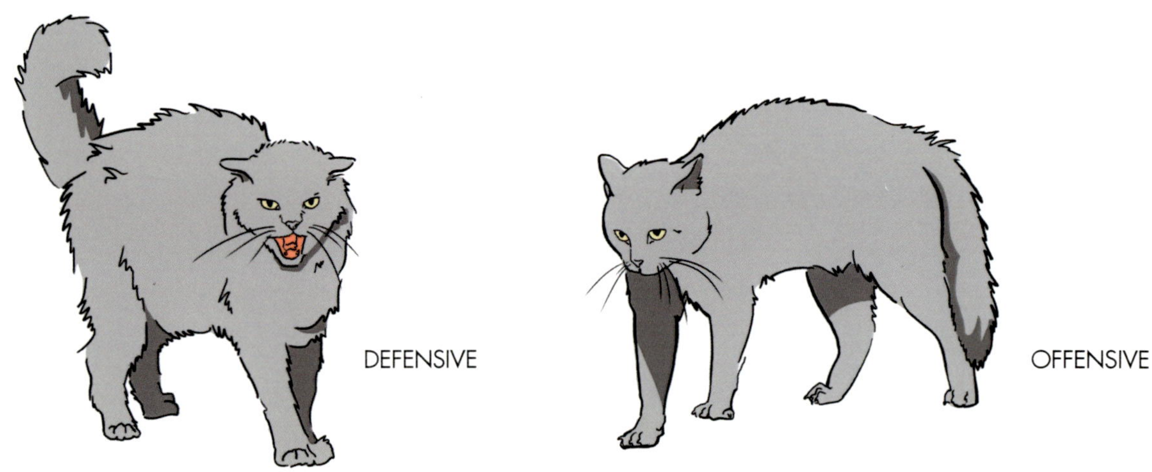

Usual postures in cats

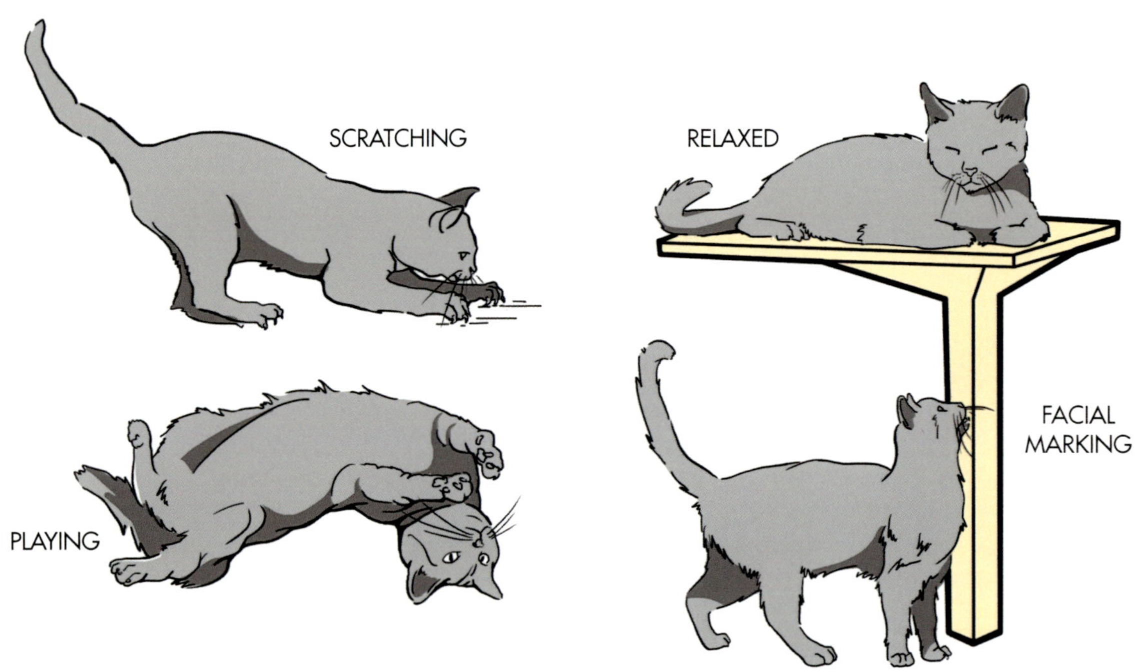

85 Neonate management

After birth, the best thing to do is to let the mother take care of her offspring. If she does not have a maternal instinct, we should immediately intervene: clear the airways and actively dry the kittens to stimulate respiration. After 24 hours, the kittens may be held with care to see their sex and ensure they are in good health. They should stay at home in a quiet place with an appropriate temperature, with their food and water bowls close to the nest.

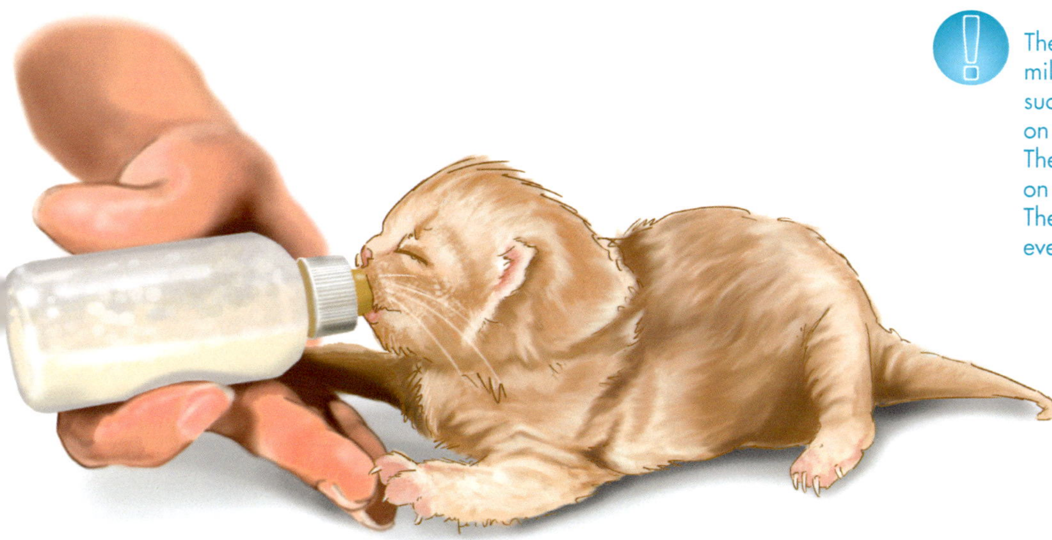

The position of the kitten when ingesting milk should be that adopted naturally when suckling on its mother, that is to say, lying on its stomach with the head stretched. The kitten should be able to put its forelimbs on the bottle teat or on the carer's hands. The feeding bottle should be washed after every use and sterilised at least once a day.

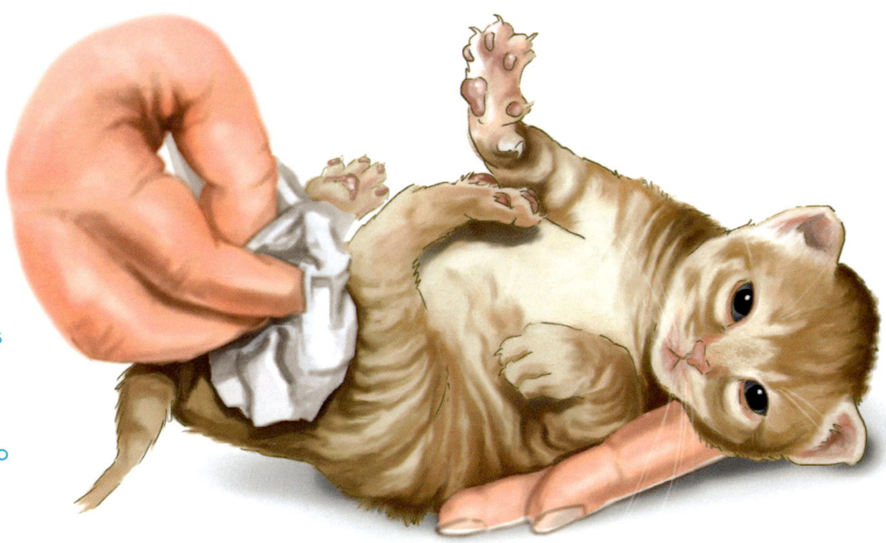

During the first 3–4 weeks of life, a gentle massage should be performed on the perianal area with a warm, damp cotton bud to stimulate micturition and defecation.

Orphaned kitten care

- Warm and constant ambient temperature (use of lamps, hot water bottles, blankets, etc.):
  - 1st week: 30–32 °C.
  - 2nd week: 26–29 °C.
  - From the 3rd week: 21–24 °C.
- Clean, comfortable place, with no air currents (e.g. box with a minimum height of 15 cm, with a towel or blanket).
- Feeding: special formula for kittens, warm (35–38 °C), administered every 2–3 hours during the first weeks of life by means of special feeding bottles or syringes (attached to a teat to prevent them from aspirating the milk).